CHROMOSOMAL VARIATION IN MAN

CHROMOSOMAL VARIATION
IN MAN
A CATALOG OF CHROMOSOMAL VARIANTS
AND ANOMALIES

Digamber S. Borgaonkar

The Johns Hopkins University Press
BALTIMORE AND LONDON

Manufactured in the United States of America

The Johns Hopkins University Press, Baltimore, Maryland 21218
The Johns Hopkins University Press Ltd., London

Library of Congress Catalog Card Number 75-10517
ISBN 0-8018-1719-6

Library of Congress Cataloging in Publication data
will be found on the last printed page of this book.

TO MY WIFE, MANDA PURANDARE BORGAONKAR

CONTENTS

LIST OF TABLES

PREFACE

During the last fifteen years human cytogeneticists have attempted to cope with the bibliographic problems that stem from rapid developments in the field. Some have collected the data and presented them in a concise form. For example, Thompson (1965, 1966) compiled the material on autosomes and provided a catalog. Hamerton (1971) and Baserga, Castoldi, and Dallapiccola (1973) have tabulated large amounts of data on abnormal karyotypes in their respective books. However, because of the rapid advances made in the techniques for studying chromosomes and the flooding of the literature with reports on all types of anomalies, a survey was likely to be out-of-date by the time it was published. A convenient and efficient system of retrieving information on abnormal karyotypes had, therefore, become necessary.

I was fortunate to have had an idea at the right time in the right places. During the first half of 1974, for part of the time, I was associated with the laboratory of Dr. Frank Ruddle, Department of Biology, in the Kline Biology Tower, Yale University, New Haven, Connecticut. While Dr. Chester Partridge and I were discussing the use of chromosomally abnormal human cell lines for regional assignment of loci in somatic cell hybridization, a question arose as to what material was available and how the information should be stored. The methodology of the catalog was conceived during the discussions I held with numerous colleagues at Yale and Johns Hopkins. I believe the *Atma** of the catalog is in this methodology of organization, its simplicity of use, and the ease and economy with which it can be updated.

The first section of the catalog deals with structural chromosomal variations and anomalies, such as deletions, inversions, and translocations. They are entered in the catalog according to the chromosome break points. The first two digits of the entry number refer to the chromosome (01 to 22, OX and OY); the third digit refers to the chromosome arms (*p* and *q*); and the fourth, fifth, and sixth digits refer to the region, band, and sub-band, respectively. Whenever information corresponding to the latter four columns is not available, a *0* is entered in the appropriate columns. If and when further information on such an entry becomes available, the revised information will be substituted. Thus, the first autosome item encoded is 010000 and the last 22q130. In other words, the minimal information required is which chromosome is involved. The break points reported in structural aberrations are entered. In general, I have adopted a policy to list almost all the recent reports of structural aberrations. The entry numbers are arranged in numerical order. Whenever each entry has information on two or more break points (or abnormalities), then at the second and succeeding entries an appropriate reference is inserted. For example, the translocation t(5;14)(p14;q21) will have its complete entry at 05p140, and its secondary entry at 14q210 will have the following notation: Same entry as in 05p140 (Borgaonkar et al. 1973).

The second section of the catalog lists numerical anomalies which include trisomies, monosomies, and polyploids. The first two digits of the entry refer to the chromosome number, while the third digit is either a minus (–) or plus (+) sign, indicat-

---

*A Sanskrit word meaning, roughly, the immortal soul or spirit of an individual.

ing monosomy or trisomy respectively. References on polyploidy are arranged in alphabetical order. In this section and, in fact, in other sections, it was found desirable not to include some earlier references, for the same type of aberration as these can be found in the bibliographies of later reports that are cited. Certain references selected on the basis of their uniqueness, priority, etc., are cited.

In a third section of the catalog I have included those disorders which are labeled "Chromosomal Breakage Syndromes." Since these disorders are presumed to be non-specific for a single chromosome they have been entered under a separate category and are listed in alphabetical order. I recognize that this is an exception to the rest of the cataloging methodology, but I included these entries so as to cover the range of chromosomal anomalies in man.

Under each entry number all the references are listed alphabetically according to the last name of the first author. The bibliographic citation is followed by chromosome constitution(s) of the individual(s) reported. To avoid confusion created by multiple reporting of the same case, the subjects are identified by their case number, when available. One of the uses of the catalog is in chromosome assignment. Therefore, it is desirable to include information on the availability of mutant cell lines. I have been fortunate in having the collaboration of Drs. Coriell and Greene of the Institute for Medical Research, Camden, New Jersey. The listings of chromosomally abnormal cell lines available in their repository are included in this catalog, along with the identifying number.

In compiling this catalog some arbitrary decisions have been necessary. Some of these may have to be reconsidered as additional data become available.

i)   If no specific break points were described in the report, but could be deciphered easily from the figures or from the contents of the paper, then the inferred break points were cataloged.

ii) From the numerous reports on relatively common conditions, such as the +13, +18, +21 trisomies, the 5p-, 18p- partial monosomies, and the 45,X and 47,XXY sex chromosomal abnormalities, only a few reports have been cataloged on the basis of priority, uniqueness, or general coverage.

iii) Reports on mosaics and chimeras, and on tumor, cancer, and leukemic cell lines have been almost completely excluded; a few significant reports on these are included.

iv) Data on experimentally produced chromosomal break points have also been excluded, but are available elsewhere (Morad, Jonasson, & Lindsten 1973).

In the catalog I have attempted to adhere, as far as possible, to the guidelines put forward by the Paris Conference (1971). However, several departures or modifications seemed appropriate:

a)   In the aneuploidy section of the catalog, I have maintained the first two digits in the entry for the chromosome number. These are followed by the designations (+) for a trisomy and (–) for a monosomy. Double aneuploidy is entered in the same manner. In this section all entries are in numerical order followed by X and Y. For multiple sex chromosomal anomalies, those of the X chromosome are listed first.

b)   In translocations where changes in length only were known, only one bracket was used, e.g., 46,XX,t(5p+;13q–). No assumption was made with regard to the reciprocal nature of translocations unless this was so stated in the report. A statement of balanced translocation in a report was not interpreted as synonymous to reciprocal translocation.

c) Whenever an existing band is subdivided, the Paris Conference (1971) called for a decimal point to be placed after the original band designation, followed by the number assigned to each sub-band. We have not used a decimal point in the entry numbers.

To facilitate collection of data on possible preferential involvement of certain chromosomal regions in aberrations, we have included, with the entry number, the banding pattern for the band or sub-band, i.e., Negative, Positive, or Variable as per the Q and G banding techniques (see Table 1). This information would be helpful in the understanding of the mechanics of aberration as we begin to understand the biochemical basis of the banding techniques. Admittedly, these figures reflect only those break points that are reported in the literature and entered into the catalog. Considerable bias goes into what the investigator considers a significant finding and what is fit for publication. The difference between the expected involvement of the three different types of band regions (negative, positive, and variable), based on their proportionate occurrence in the genome, and the actual, observed in the break points, was statistically significant.

Besides the reason stated earlier, we thought that there were other significant reasons for undertaking a computerized chromosomal catalog:

1. The geneticist may pool linkage data obtained by the pedigree approach using marker chromosomes. The catalog could be used in the selection of cell lines for regional assignment of loci by the somatic cell hybridization approach.

2. In the description of new clinical material with chromosomal abnormalities, it is becoming difficult to ascertain from the vast body of literature, what, if anything, has been published before on the same type of chromosome abnormality. The information that is available in abstracting journals is not easily culled. It is hoped that with the aid of this catalog such a need will be easily met.

3. Individuals not wishing to report formally an abnormal karyotype may elect to report it in this catalog as a personal communication. In due course, a sufficient experience with a particular abnormality may accumulate that the authors can join forces in a formal report.

4. In structural aberrations it will be possible to relate the involvement of a particular type of band to the proportionate occurrence of that type of band in the human karyotype. We can also relate the type of abnormality to these regions.

5. We have categorized the chromosomal anomalies and variations into 20 groups (Table 2). Since these are, in effect, written into the main body of the catalog, we have chosen to code them. These anomalies and variations as found for the different chromosomes are tabulated. This will facilitate compilation of data on the various

Table 1. Band Region and Break Points

	Break points		Proportion in the genome*
Band region	Number of entries	Percentage	
Negative	450	64.4	47.6
Positive	101	14.4	46.7
Variable	148	21.2	6.1
Total	699	100	

*Calculated as per the diagrammatic representation of chromosome bands in Figure 5 of the Paris Conference (1971).

Table 2. Abberation Code

No.	Code	Description	No.	Code	Description
1.	IC	Isochromosome	11.	II	Inverted insertion within a chromosome
2.	TD	Terminal deletion	12.	IX	Direct insertion between two chromosomes
3.	ID	Interstitial deletion			
4.	IP	Inversion paracentric	13.	XI	Inverted insertion between two chromosomes
5.	PI	Pericentric inversion			
6.	RI	Ring chromosome	14.	CT	Complex translocation
7.	DI	Dicentric chromosome	15.	FT	Four-break translocation
8.	RT	Reciprocal translocation	16.	ST	Simple translocation
9.	TR	Robertsonian translocation	17.	DU	Duplication
10.	IN	Direct insertion within a chromosome	18.	TX	Tandem translocation
			19.	RE	Recombinant chromosome
			20.	MA	Marker chromosome

For the sake of convenience, explanations of the above terms are provided here. For details the reader should consult standard textbooks on cytogenetics.

Isochromosome: The two arms of the chromosome are identical to one another.

Terminal deletion: A terminal segment of a chromosome is deleted.

Interstitial deletion: An intermediary segment, i.e., excluding a centromere and terminal ends (telomeres), of a chromosome is deleted.

Inversion paracentric: An inversion of chromosome segment that does not include the centromere.

Pericentric inversion: An inversion of a chromosome segment that includes the centromere.

Ring chromosome: When two broken ends of a chromosome have joined to form a ring-like structure.

Dicentric chromosome: A chromosome with two centromeres.

Reciprocal translocation: In a translocation the segments of chromosomes have been exchanged.

Robertsonian translocation: When the translocation involves the acrocentric chromosomes, e.g., 13 and 21.

Direct insertion within a chromosome: When a segment has been inserted in the same chromosome at another point.

Inverted insertion within a chromosome: When the segment that has been inserted in the same chromosome at another point is inverted in relation to the centromere.

Direct insertion between two chromosomes: When a segment from one chromosome has been inserted at a point in another chromosome.

Inverted insertion between two chromosomes: When the segment from one chromosome that has been inserted at a point in another chromosome has been inverted in its relationship to the centromere.

Complex translocation: A translocation involving three or more chromosomes (refer to Paris Conference [1971], p. 31, for further details).

Four-break translocation: A double reciprocal translocation (refer to Paris Conference [1971], pp. 31–34, for further details).

Simple translocation: A transfer of a segment of one chromosome to another.

Duplication: A chromosome in which a segment is present in duplicate.

Tandem translocation: A transfer of a segment of one chromosome to another at the end of its arm.

Recombinant chromosome: A structurally rearranged chromosome with a new segmental composition resulting from meiotic crossing over between a displaced segment and its normally located counterpart in certain types of structural counterparts.

Marker chromosome: This term has been rather loosely used here so as to include any chromosome with a polymorphic or variant feature.

types of abnormalities that occur in specific chromosomes, e.g., which of the 24 human chromosomes occur as ring chromosomes or as isochromosomes. Table 3 lists these aberrations vis-à-vis the chromosome number.

6. It is my intent to adapt the method of the catalog to establish an International Registry of Abnormal Karyotypes. It would then, for example, be possible to make inferences about the prevalence rate of chromosomal abnormalities.

7. Since the data on abnormal karyotypes will be assembled, it should be possible to work on the problems related to the estimation of risk in the transmission of ab-

Table 3. Numbers of Different Aberrations as They Were Found in the Catalog for the Various Human Chromosomes

Chromosome Number	Aberration																			
	IC	TD	ID	IP	PI	RI	DI	RT	TR	IN	II	IX	XI	CT	FT	ST	DU	TX	RE	MA
1	0	4	1	0	5	2	0	6	0	2	2	0	0	3	1	42	0	0	0	8
2	0	0	1	0	6	0	0	5	0	0	1	1	0	1	0	39	1	2	0	4
3	0	0	0	0	9	1	0	3	0	0	0	2	1	0	0	21	0	0	0	2
4	0	15	0	0	5	5	0	5	0	1	0	1	0	0	0	30	0	0	0	0
5	0	10	1	0	5	4	1	6	0	0	0	1	0	1	0	18	0	0	0	0
6	0	1	0	0	1	2	0	5	0	0	0	0	0	1	0	14	1	1	0	0
7	0	0	0	0	1	2	0	4	0	0	0	0	0	1	0	12	0	0	0	0
8	0	2	1	0	5	1	0	4	0	0	0	1	0	0	0	8	0	0	0	0
9	0	3	0	0	7	3	0	12	0	0	0	0	0	0	0	25	0	0	0	6
10	0	0	0	0	1	1	0	5	0	0	0	0	0	0	0	5	0	0	1	0
11	0	1	0	0	1	0	0	3	0	0	0	1	1	1	0	13	0	0	0	0
12	0	2	0	0	0	1	2	0	0	0	0	0	0	0	0	3	0	1	0	0
13	1	6	1	0	4	13	3	4	30	0	0	1	0	0	0	4	2	1	0	3
14	0	1	0	0	0	1	1	1	8	0	0	0	0	0	0	11	0	0	0	2
15	0	5	0	0	3	2	1	1	7	0	0	0	0	0	0	5	0	0	0	9
16	0	0	1	1	0	0	0	0	0	0	0	0	0	0	0	3	0	0	0	6
17	0	1	0	0	0	1	0	0	0	0	0	0	0	0	0	5	0	0	0	8
18	2	11	0	0	1	7	0	5	0	0	0	0	0	0	0	19	1	1	0	0
19	0	1	0	0	2	1	0	0	0	0	0	0	0	0	0	4	0	0	0	0
20	0	0	0	0	0	2	0	1	1	0	0	0	0	0	0	0	0	0	0	0
21	1	4	0	0	0	6	1	0	12	0	0	0	0	0	0	2	0	5	0	7
22	0	6	0	0	0	5	1	0	0	0	0	0	0	0	0	2	0	1	0	6
X	11	13	0	0	1	1	2	3	0	0	0	0	0	0	0	37	1	4	0	1
Y	4	8	0	0	11	6	5	0	1	0	0	0	0	0	0	16	0	0	0	13

normal rearrangements and involvement of factors such as sex and bias of ascertainment.

A catalog such as this probably would not have been meaningful prior to the significant advances made in karyotyping the chromosomes of man. The "banding" techniques not only enabled us to know more about the nature and extent of variations and anomalies but also helped to define the chromosome regions (Paris Conference, 1971). The incidence of chromosomal variations and anomalies in liveborns seems to be in the vicinity of 5% and in zygotes is several times more than this figure. Prior to the advent of banding techniques it was thought that there were several chromosomes which are "spared" from involvement in aberrations, partly because of the nature of genetic material present on them. I have shown elsewhere (Borgaonkar, in press) that each and every chromosome has now been implicated in interchanges. It appears that now we can extend this approach to determine whether each and every arm, region, and band of each chromosome is involved in producing variation.

December 1974   D. S. B.

REFERENCES:

Baserga, A., Castoldi, G. L., and Dallapiccola, B. *La Patologia Cromosomica.* Rome: Edizioni L. Pozzi, 1973.

Borgaonkar, D. S. Autosomal abnormalities and the banding techniques. In *Modern Trends in Human Genetics.* Ed. A. E. H. Emery. London: Butterworth Ltd., in press.

Hamerton, J. L. *Human Cytogenetics.* 2 vols. New York: Academic Press, 1971.

McKusick, V. A. *Mendelian Inheritance in Man.* 4th edition. Baltimore: The Johns Hopkins University Press, 1975.

Morad, M., Jonasson, J., and Lindsten, J. "Distribution of mitomycin C induced breaks on human chromosomes." *Hereditas* 74: 273–82 (1973).

Paris Conference (1971). *Standardization in Human Cytogenetics.* Birth Defects: Original Article Series, VIII: 7. New York: The National Foundation, 1972.

Thompson, H. "Abnormalities of the autosomal chromosomes associated with human disease. Selected topics and catalogues." *Amer. J. Med. Sci.* 250: 718–34 (1965), and 251: 706–35 (1966).

ON THE USE OF THE CATALOG

There are certain modifications in style because of the computer usage. Special characters from foreign languages, such as French accents and the German umlaut, could not be reproduced.

In the catalog the entry numbers are arranged numerically. The first two digits refer to the chromosome numbers, the third digit refers to the chromosomes arm, and the fourth, fifth, and sixth digits refer to the region, band, and sub-bands, according to the conventions recommended by the Paris Conference (1971) nomenclature.

An author index has been provided which may facilitate location of a report; sometimes it is easier to remember the individuals reporting an abnormality rather than the specifics of the report. I have provided on each page a picture of the relevant chromosome from Figure 5 of the Paris Conference (1971). This will, I am sure, be of help in the understanding of the chromosome region that is being discussed on that page.

I have taken the liberty of changing the initials of some authors so as to have uniformity in their names; for example, Newton, M., and Newton, M.S., are one and the same person, but appeared differently in reports.

The following errors in the catalog have come to my attention too late for correction in the text:

On page 46, line 6, the following information should appear:

Same entry as in 01q200 (Neu and Gardner, 1973).

The following heading should be inserted on page 96, line 12:

12p120   Positive band.

The listing for K. Boczkowski and M. Mikkelsen on page 168 should precede the entries for D. S. Borgaonkar on page 167, immediately following the heading "OXp110   Negative band."

C. Palmer and C. G. Palmer, given as separate entries in the author index, should be combined, since both refer to the same person.

Dr. Hirschhorn's name was unintentionally omitted from references to works by M. Lucas and I. Wallace, of which he is co-author, on pages 7, 57, 87, and 150.

The names of J. Halbfass and Souvatzoglou (no initals), listed in the entry for Zang, Singer, et al., on page 166, were inadvertently omitted from the author index.

SOURCES

In compiling these catalogs I was benefited by the availability of a reprint file that I have maintained over the years. I am most grateful to various colleagues who sent their reprints.

The *Current Contents* was useful in keeping up with the literature.

The following journals were surveyed for entries since 1970: *American Journal of Human Genetics, Annales de Génétique, Annals of Human Genetics, Clinical Genetics, Cytogenetics and Cell Genetics, Humangenetik, Human Heredity*, and *Journal of Medical Genetics.*

A check with *Excerpta Medica* (abstracts on Human Genetics) and *Index Medicus* was valuable for some of the reports from earlier years.

I have included a few reports as personal communications and as unpublished observations of our own. The number of such reports may increase significantly, since many chromosome abnormalities remain unpublished but may be worth documenting in a catalog such as this. In fact, if the documentation of several similar abnormalities reveals significant leads, the authors of personal communications may be encouraged to report them in full. I would welcome personal communications from colleagues. There are several citations entitled "Rotterdam Conference (1974)" in this catalog. No further information has been provided as the proceedings of this conference are to be published by The National Foundation–March of Dimes, New York, in their Birth Defects: Original Article Series. It was the Second International Workshop on Human Gene Mapping. Furthermore, since I have no pretense to infallibility in the collation and interpretation of the published data, I would welcome having errors and omissions called to my attention.

ACKNOWLEDGMENTS

David Bolling and his staff in the computer laboratory (especially Deborah Holifield) have been responsible for the programming and other related matters. As stated earlier, I have benefited in the development of this catalog from the numerous discussions that I have had with Dr. Victor A. McKusick, the members of the Division of Medical Genetics at Johns Hopkins University, and the staff of the laboratory of Dr. Frank H. Ruddle at Yale University. The mechanics of computerization of the catalog is similar to that followed by Dr. McKusick for his *Mendelian Inheritance in Man*, and I benefited from the fact that that was also a product of the same department. Helen Cutler generously devoted much of her time keying in the data on the magnetic tape.

Several students, assistants, and post-doctoral fellows have been helpful (in particular, Eric Starr and Sue Blair) in going over many details. However, I take the responsibility for any omissions and errors. I would appreciate being informed about those which may have been overlooked and still appear here. It will be possible to correct entries or add new ones on the tape, since we propose to update this catalog continuously.

Financial support for this catalog came from a Genetics Center Grant of the United States Public Health Service, GM 19489, and from NIH contract NO1 GM-3-2112 and a grant from The National Foundation-March of Dimes, New York.

CHROMOSOMAL VARIATION IN MAN

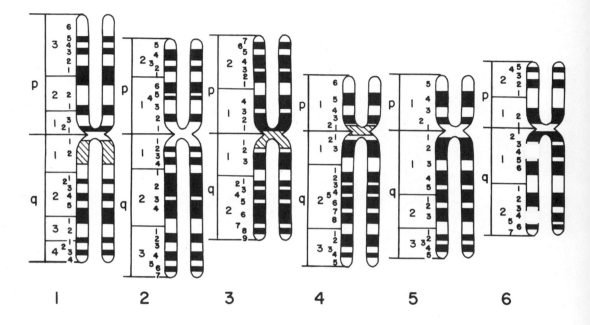

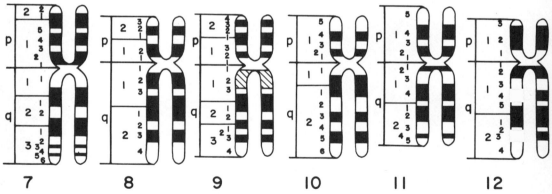

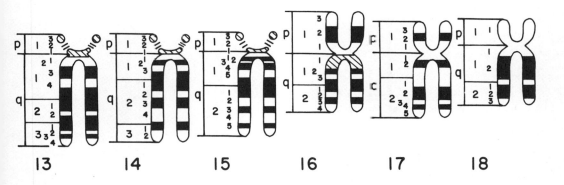

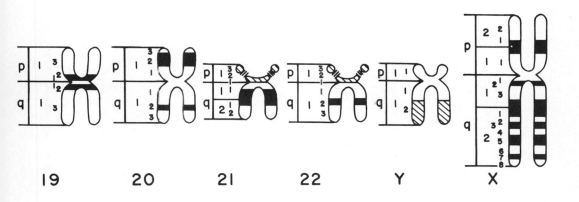

Modified diagrammatic representation of chromosome bands, as adapted from Figure 5 of *Standardization in Human Cytogenetics*, Birth Defects: Original Article Series, VIII: 7 (New York: The National Foundation, 1972).

STRUCTURAL VARIATIONS AND ANOMALIES

0 10000

Craig-Holmes, A. P., Moore, F. B. and Shaw, M.
W.: Polymorphism of human C-band heterochroma-
tin. I. Frequency of variants. Amer. J. Hum.
Genet. 25:181-192, 1973.

Kontras, S. B., Currier, G. J., Cooper, R. F. and
Ambuel, J. P.: Maternal transmission of a 21/1
translocation associated with Down's syndrome.
J. Pediat. 69:635-639, 1966.
46,XX,t(1;21)(?;q).
46,XX and XY,der(1)der(21)t(1;21)(?;q)mat.
47,XX,der(1)der(21)t(1;21)(?;q)mat,+21.

Robson, E. B., Polani, P. E., Dart, S. J.,
Jacobs, P. A. and Renwick, J. H.: Probable
assignment of the alpha locus of haptoglobin to
chromosome 16 in man. Nature 223:1163-1165,
1969.
46,XX and XY,t(1-;16+).
46,XX and XY,der(1)der(16)t(1-;16+)mat and pat.

Surana, R. B., Conen, P. E., Brando, M. and
Keith, J. D.: Familial tertiary trisomy with
t(14q-;1+?). Birth Defects: Original Article
Series X(No.8):53-65, 1974.
Cases S.R. and M.V. in this report.
46,XY,+t(14q-;1+?).
46,XX and XY,der(1)der(14)t(14q-;1+?)mat and pat.

Thompson, H.: Familial chromosomal translocation
with distinctive phenotype due to effective
trisomy of No. 11p. Newport Beach, Calif., Birth
Defects Conf., National Foundation - March of
Dimes, p. 88, June 16-21, 1974.
46,XX,t(1;11)(?;p11).
46,XX,t(1;11)(1qter to 1pter::11p11 to
11pter;11qter to 11p1:).
46,XX,-1,der(1)t(1;11)(?;p11)mat.
46,XX,-1,der(1)t(1;11)(1qter to 1pter::11p11 to
11pter)mat.
The author implies that only one break occurred
to form the translocation chromosome.

01p000

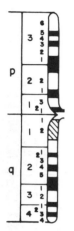

Bhasin, M. K., Foerster, W. and Fuhrmann, W.: A cytogenetic study of recurrent abortion. Humangenetik 18:139-148, 1973.
Case 2 (J. No. 531-72) in this report.
46,XX,inv(1)(pq).

Buckton, K. E.: The identification of whole chromosomes or parts of chromosomes by the new banding techniques. Nobel Symposium 23:196-200, 1972.
46,XX,t(1p-;3p+),t(3q-;9q+).
See also 01p320 (Jacobs et al., 1974).

Ebbin, A. J., Wilson, M. G., Towner, J. W. and Forsman, I.: An inherited 1/G translocation. J. Med. Genet. 8:536-539, 1971.
46,XX,t(1?;G)(p;q)/47,XX,t(1?;G)(p;q),+mar.

Francke, U.: Quinacrine mustard fluorescence of human chromosomes: characterization of unusual translocations. Amer. J. Hum. Genet. 24:189-213, 1972.
Case No. I.E.C. 082963 in this report.
46,XX,t(1;13)(p;p1),22p-.

Gray, J. E., Syrett, J. E., Ritchie, K. M. and Elliott, W. D.: An interstitial translocation: chromosome No. 1p to 4q. Lancet 2:92-93, 1972.
46,XX,inv ins(4;1)(q2;p1 or 2 or 3).
The authors hypothesize that the small terminal region (1pter to 1p3 of chromosome No. 1) has been lost.

Kyaosaar, M. E.: A study of chromosomes in couples with habitual abortions. Genetika 7:117-121, 1971 and Soviet Genetics 7:1600-1603, 1974.
46,XX,t(1p-;Gq+).

Lubs, H. A. and Lubs, M. L.: Studies of newborns in Grand Junction, Colorado. Twelfth Ann. Somatic Cell Genet. Conf. Utah, 78-79, 1974.
46,XX,t(1p+;4q-).

Mikelsaar, A. V. N., Ananjev, E. V. and Gindilis, V. M.: Probable pericentric inversion in chromosome No. 1 in a female child (46,XX,inv(1p+q-)). Humangenetik 9:316-324. 1970.
46,XX,inv(1).

Newton, M. S., Cunningham, C., Jacobs, P. A., Price, W. H. and Fraser, I. A.: Chromosome survey of a hospital for the mentally subnormal. Part 2: Autosome abnormalities. Clin. Genet. 3:226-248. 1972.
M. R. C. Registry No. K137-18-67 in this report.
46,XY,t(1p-;13q+).
See also 01p130 (Jacobs et al., 1974).

Seleznev, Y. V. and Dzenis, I. G.: Longitudinal differentiation of human mitotic chromosomes. Communication II. Analysis of pericentric inversion of the first chromosome in a child with anomalous sex differentiation. Genetika 8:115-119, 1972.
46,XY/47,XXY,inv(1)(pq).

Sharma, G. and Sobti, R. C.: A case with 46,XY,1r-46,XY,A-,C+, chromosomal constitution. Mammalian Chromosome Newsletter 15:21, 1974.
46,XY,r(1).

Wolf, C. B., Peterson, J. A., LoGrippo, G. A. and Weiss, L.: Ring 1 chromosome and dwarfism - a possible syndrome. J. Pediat. 71:719-722, 1967.
46,XX,r(1).

01p130   Negative band

Jacobs, P. A., Buckton, K. E., Cunningham, C. and Newton, M. S.: An analysis of the break points of structural rearrangements in man. J. Med. Genet. 11:50-64, 1974.
M. R. C. Registry No. K137-18-67 in this report.
46,XY,t(1;13)(p13;q22).

Lee, C. S. N., Ying, K. L. and Bowen, P.: Position of the Duffy locus on chromosome 1 in relation to breakpoints for structural rearrangements. Amer. J. Hum. Genet. 26:93-102, 1974.
46,XX,inv(1)(p13q23).
46,XX,inv(1)(pter to p13::q23 to p13::q23 to qter).

01p210   Positive band

Brown, J. A. and Shows, T. B.: Rotterdam Conference, 1974.

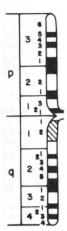

46,XX,t(1;2)(p21;q37).
46,XX,t(1;2)(1qter to 1p21::2q37 to 2qter;2pter to 2q37::1p21 to 1pter).

Shows, T. B. and Brown, J. A.: A 1;2 transloca-tion facilitates the assignment and regional mapping of eight enzyme loci on chromosomes 1 and 2 in somatic cell hybrids. Amer. J. Hum. Genet. 26:80A, 1974.
46,XX,t(1;2)(p21;q37).

Sutherland, G. R., Bauld, R. and Bain, A. D.: Observations on human amniotic fluid cell strains in serial culture. J. Med. Genet. 11:190-195, 1974.
46,XY,t(1;12)(p21;q21).

01p300

Nuzzo, F., Giorgi, R., Zuffardi, O. and Dambro-sio, F.: Translocation t(1p+;2q-) associated with recurrent abortion. Ann. Genet. 16:211-214, 1973.
46,XX,t(1;2)(p3;q1).

Tartaglia, A. P., Propp, S., Amarose, A. P., Propp, R. P. and Hall, C. A.: Chromosome abnor-mality and hypocalcemia in congenital erythroid hypoplasia (blackfan-diamond syndrome). Amer. J. Med. 41:990-999, 1966.
A gap was reported in this region.

01p320   Negative band

de la Chapelle, A.: Personal communication, 1973.
47,XX,+21,t(1;17)(p32;p13).
47,XX,+21,t(1;17)(1pter to 1p32::17p13 to 17qter;17pter to 17p13::1p32 to 1qter).
Mutant Cell Repository No. GM-201.

Jacobs, P. A., Buckton, K. E., Cunningham, C. and Newton, M. S.: An analysis of the break points of structural rearrangements in man. J. Med. Genet. 11:50-64, 1974.
M. R. C. Registry No. K42-352-67 in this report.
46,XY,t(1;16)(p32;q22).
M. R. C. Registry No. K118-119-68 in this report.

46,XY,t(1;16)(p32;q24).
M. R. C. Registry No. K180-48-68 in this report.
46,XX,t(1;13)(3;9)(p32;p25 or 26 or 27q21;q22).
M. R. C. Registry No. K212-171-72 in this report.
46,XX,inv(1)(p32q42).
46,XX,inv(1)(pter to p32::q42 to p32::q42 to qter).

Marsh, W. L., Chaganti, R. S. K., Gardner, F. H., Mayer, K., Nowell, P. C. and German, J.: Mapping human autosomes: Evidence supporting assignment of Rhesus to the short arm of chromosome No. 1. Science 183:966-968, 1974.
See 04q310, 07q110 and 07q320, del(1)(qter to p33:).

01p330   Positive band

Douglas, G. R., McAlpine, P. J. and Hamerton, J. L.: Regional localization of loci for human PGM1 and 6PGD on human chromosome one by use of hybrids of Chinese hamster/human somatic cells. Proc. Natl. Acad. Sci., USA, 70:2737-2740, 1973.
Hybrid clone with del(1)(p33 to pter).

Pan, S. F., Fatora, S. R., Garver, K. L. and Steele, M. W.: Meiotic consequences of heterozygosis for a homologous insertion into chromosome #1. Amer. J. Hum. Genet. 26:65A, 1974.
46,XY,ins(1)(p33q32q43).
This familial insertion was found in three generations with duplications and deficiencies.

01p360   Negative band

Hecht, F.: Personal Communication, 1974.
46,XY,t(1;15)(p36;q1).
Mutant Cell Repository No. GM-126.

Lozzio, C. B. and Klepper, M. B.: Chromosome aberrations identified by the new banding techniques. Amer. J. Hum. Genet. 26:55A, 1974.
ins(1)(p36q21q25).
This familial insertion is reported here.

Steffensen, D. M.: Rotterdam Conference, 1974.
t(1;15)(p36;q14).

01q000

Same entry as in 01p000 (Bhasin, Foerster and Fuhrmann, 1973).

Buckton, K. E.: The identification of whole chromosomes or parts of chromosomes by the new banding techniques. Nobel Symposium 23:196-200, 1972.
46,XX,t(1q+;14q-).

Chandley, A. C. and Fletcher, J. M.: Centromere staining in man. Humangenetik 18:247-252, 1973.
46,XY,t(1;18)(q;q).
46,XY,t(1;18)(1pter to 1q::18q to 18qter;18pter to 18q::1qter to qter).

Ferguson-Smith, M. A.: Rotterdam Conference, 1974.
t(1q;5q).

Jacobs, P. A., Brunton, M., Frackiewicz, A., Newton, M. S., Cook, P. J. L. and Robson, E. B.: Studies on a family with three cytogenetic markers. Ann. Hum. Genet. 33:325-336, 1970.
46,XY,t(1q;Cq-).

Leisti, J.: Structural variation in human mitotic chromosomes. Ann. Acad. Sci. fenn. (Med.) Series A, IV, Biologica 179:1-69, 1971.
46,XY,t(1q-;5p+).
Case No. 21 in this report.
46,XY,-5+der(5)t(1q-;5p+)pat.

Maganias, N. H., Archambault, L., Becker, K. L. and Winnacker, J. L.: A 1-G translocation in a member of a kindred with a marker chromosome. Arch. Int. Med. 119:297-301, 1967.
46,XX,t(1q-;Gq+).

Therkelsen, A. J., Petersen, G. B., Steenstrup, O. R., Jonasson, J., Lindsten, J. and Zech, L.: Prenatal diagnosis of chromosome abnormalities. Acta Paediat. Scand. 61:397-404, 1972.
46,XY,t(1;22)(q;q1).
Case No. 93 in this report.
46,XY,der(1)der(22)t(1;22)(q;q1)pat.

van den Berghe, H., van Eygen, M., Fryns, J. P., Tanghe, W. and Verresen, H.: Partial trisomy 1, karyotype 46,XY,12-,t(1q,12p)+. Humangenetik 18:225-230, 1973.
46,XX,t(1;12)(q;p1).
46,XY,-12,+der(12)t(1;12)(q;p1)mat.
46,XY,-12,+der(12)t(1;12)(12qter to 12p1::1q to 1qter)mat.

01q110   Negative band

Hirschhorn, K., Lucas, M. and Wallace, I.: Precise identification of various chromosomal abnormalities. Ann. Hum. Genet. 36:375-379, 1973.
Family Gr(GC641) in this report.
46,XX,t(1;13)(q11;p11).
46,XX,t(1;13)(1pter to 1q11::13p1⁻ to 13pter;13qter to 13p11::1q11 to 1qter).

Lucas, M. and Wallace, I.: Recurrent abortions and chromosome abnormalities. J. Obstet. Gynaec. Brit. Comm. 79:1119-1127, 1972.
Family Gr in this report.
46,XX,t(1;13)(q11;p11).
46,XX,t(1;13)(1pter to 1q11::13p1⁻ to 13pter;13qter to 13p11::1q11 to 1qter).

01q120   Variable band

Cooper, H. L. and Hernits, R.: A familial chromosome variant in a subject with anomalous sex differentiation. Amer. J. Hum. Genet. 15:465-475, 1963.

Donahue, R. P., Bias, W. B., Renwick, J. H. and McKusick, V. A.: Probable assignment of the duffy blood group locus to chromosome 1 in man. Proc. Natl. Acad. Sci., USA, 61:949-955, 1968.
46,XX, and XY,1qh+.

Friedrich, U. and Nielsen, J.: Autosomal reciprocal translocations in newborn children and their relatives. Humangenetik 21:133-144, 1974.
46,XX,t(1;16)(q12;q12).
46,XX,t(1;16)(1pter to 1q12::16q12 to 16qter;16pter to 16q12::1q12 to 1qter).
46,XX and XY,der(1)der(16)t(1;16)(q12;q12)mat.

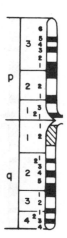

Proband No. 5030 in this report.
46,XY,der(1)der(16)t(1;16)(q12;q12)mat.
46,XY,t(1;17)(q12;q25).
46,XY,t(1;17)(1pter to 1q12::17q25 to 17qter;17pter to 17q25::1q12 to 1qter).
46,XY,der(1)der(17)t(1;17)(q12;q25)pat.
Proband No. 9062 in this report.
46,XY,der(1)der(17)t(1;17)(q12;q25)pat.

Geraedts, J. and Pearson, P. L.: Specific staining of the human No. 1 chromosome in spermatozoa. Humangenetik 20:171-173, 1973.

Holzer, A. and Rosenkranz, W.: Homozygous duplication on long arm of chromosome pair no. 1. Humangenetik 16:341-343, 1972.
46,XX and XY,1qh+.

Jacobs, P. A., Buckton, K. E., Cunningham, C. and Newton, M. S.: An analysis of the break points of structural rearrangements in man. J. Med. Genet. 11:50-64, 1974.
M. R. C. Registry No. K51-158-68 in this report.
46,XY,t(1;17)(q12;q21).

Mikelsaar, A. V. N., Tuur, S. J. and Kyaosaar, M. E.: Human karyotype polymorphism. I. Routine and fluorescence microscopic investigation of chromosomes in a normal adult population. Humangenetik 20:89-101, 1973.

Nielsen, J., Friedrich, U. and Hreidarsson, A. B.: Frequency and genetic effect of 1qh+. Humangenetik 21:193-196, 1974.

Palmer, C. G., Wang, L. Y., Rivas, M. L., Conneally, P. M. and Meyers, D.: Preferential segregation of 1qh+ variants? Amer. J. Hum. Genet. 26:65A, 1974.

Same entry as in 0Xq260 (Punnett et al., 1974).

Ying, K. L. and Ives, E. J.: Asymmetry of chromosome number 1 pair in three generations of a phenotypically normal family. Canad. J. Genet. Cytol. 10:577-589, 1968.

01q200

Same entry as in 0Xq200 (Dutrillaux, 1972).

Jacobs, P. A., Buckton, K. E., Cunningham, C. and
Newton, M. S.: An analysis of the break points
of structural rearrangements in man. J. Med.
Genet. 11:50-64, 1974.
M. R. C. Registry No. K216-231-72 in this report.
46,XX,t(1;15)(q2;q15 or q21 or q22).

Neu, R. L. and Gardner, L. I.: A partial trisomy
of chromosome 1 in a family with a t(1q-;4q+)
translocation. Clin. Genet. 4:474-479, 1973.
46,XX,t(1;4)(q2;q3).
46,XX,t(1;4)(1pter to 1q2;4pter to 4q3::1q2 to
1qter).

01q210   Negative band

Friedrich, U. and Nielsen, J.: Autosomal reciprocal translocations in newborn children and
their relatives. Humangenetik 21:133-144, 1974.
Proband No. 8700 in this report.
46,XY,t(1;17)(q21;q21).
46,XY,t(1;17)(1pter to 1q21::17q2⁻ to 17qter;17p-
ter to 17q21::1q21 to 1qter).
46,XY,der(1)der(17)t(1;17)(q21;q2⁻)pat.

Jacobs, P. A., Buckton, K. E., Cunningham, C. and
Newton, M. S.: An analysis of the break points
of structural rearrangements in man. J. Med.
Genet. 11:50-64, 1974.
M. R. C. Registry No. K3-135-61 in this report.
46,XX,t(1;11)(q21;q13).
M. R. C. Registry No. K91-135-65 in this report.
46,XY,t(1;16)(q21;p13).

Same entry as in 01p360 (Lozzio and Klepper,
1974).

01q230   Negative band

Dewald, G. W., Spurbeck, J. and Gordon, H.:
Automated videodensitometric analysis of autosomal translocations. Amer. J. Hum. Genet.
26:26A, 1974.
Family C in this report.
46,XY/46,XY,t(1;6)(q23;q?36).
There probably is a misprint here as there is no

region 3 in q arm of chromosome 6.

Same entry as in 01p130 (Lee, Ying and Bowen, 1974)

01q240   Positive band

Crandall, B. F. and Falk, R. E.: Craniosynostosis, profound growth retardation, unusual facies, and multiple minor anomalies associated with intercalary deletion: 46,XX,del(1)(q24,q31). Amer. J. Hum. Genet. 26:23A, 1974.
46,XX,del(1)(q24,q31).
46,XX,del(1)(pter to q24::q31 to qter).

01q250   Negative band

Same entry as in 01p360 (Lozzio and Klepper, 1974).

01q300

Seabright, M.: The use of proteolytic enzymes for the mapping of structural rearrangements in the chromosomes of man. Chromosoma 36:204-210, 1972.
46,XX,t(1;18)(q3; q22).
46,XY,-18,+der(18)t(1;18)(q3; q22)mat.
46,XY,-18,+der(18)t(1;18)(18pter to 18q22::1q3 to 1qter)mat.

01q310   Positive band

Same entry as in 01q240 (Crandall and Falk, 1974).

01q320   Negative band

Alfi, O. S.: Personal communication, 1973.
46,XX,t(1;2)(q32;p25).
Mutant Cell Repository No. GM-257.

Chandley, A. C., Christie, S., Fletcher, J. M., Frackiewicz, A. and Jacobs, P. A.: Translocation heterozygosity and associated subfertility in man. Cytogenetics 11:516-533, 1972.
Patient J. U. (M. R. C. Registry No. K187-288-71) in this report.

46,XY,t(1;18) (q32;q21).
46,XX and XY,der(1)der(18)t(1;18) (q32;q21)pat.

Desroches, G. A., Bradshaw, C. L. and Jones, O.
W.: A balanced reciprocal chromosomal translocation in three generations. Ann. Intern. Med.
79:407-410, 1973.
46,XY,t(1;2) (q32;q13).
46,XY,t(1;2) (1pter to 1q32::2q13 to 2qter;2pter
to 2q13::1q32 to 1qter).
46,XX and XY,der(1)der(2)t(1;2) (q32;q13)pat.

Francke, U.: Regional mapping of human MDH-1 and
IDH-1 on chromosome 2, LDHA on chromosome 11, and
thymidine kinase on chromosome 17. Amer. J. Hum.
Genet. 26:31A, 1974.
46,XY,t(1;2) (q32;13).
46,XY,t(1pter to 1q32::2q13 to 2qter;2pter to
2q13::1q32 to 1qter).

Jacobs, P. A., Buckton, K. E., Cunningham, C. and
Newton, M. S.: An analysis of the break points
of structural rearrangments in man. J. Med.
Genet. 11:50-64, 1974.
M. R. C. Registry No. K187-238-71 in this report.
46,XX,t(1;18) (q32;q21).

Same entry as in 01p330 (Pan et al., 1974).

Sanger, R., Alfi, O. S. and Donnell, G. N.:
Partial trisomy 1q in 3 patients. Amer. J. Hum.
Genet. 26:75A, 1974.
46,XX,t(1;2) (q32;p25).
Two children had partial trisomy for 1q, i.e.,
der(2)t(1;2) (q32;p25)mat.

Same entry as in 0Xq260 (Sanger, Alfi and Donnell, 1974).

Steffensen, D. M.: Rotterdam Conference, 1974.
t(1;13) (q32;q34).

01q400

Breg, W. R., Miller, D. A., Allderdice, P. W. and
Miller, O. J.: Identification of translocation
chromosomes by quinacrine fluorescence. Amer. J.
Dis. Child. 123:561-564, 1972.

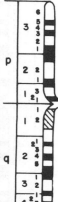

46,XX,t(1;18)(q4;p11).
Patient No. 6 in this report.
46,XX and XY,-18,+der(18)t(1;18)(q4;p11)mat.

01q420   Negative band

de la Chapelle, A.:   1974.
46,XY,del(1)(q42).
46,XY,del(1)(pter to q42:).
Mutant Cell Repository No. GM-214.

Jacobs, P. A., Buckton, K. E., Cunningham, C. and
Newton, M. S.: An analysis of the break points
of structural rearrangements in man. J. Med.
Genet. 11:50-64, 1974.
M. R. C. Registry No. K90-233-70 in this report.
46,XY,t(1;14)(q42;q23).

Same entry as in 01p320 (Jacobs et al., 1974).

01q430   Positive band

Jacobs, P. A., Buckton, K. E., Cunningham, C. and
Newton, M. S.: An analysis of the break points
of structural rearrangements in man. J. Med.
Genet. 11:50-64, 1974.
M. R. C. Registry No. K26-82-66 in this report.
46,XY,t(1;11)(q43;q21).

Martinetti, J. and Noel, B.: Remaniement complexe de novo touchant quatre chromosomes chez un
nouveau-ne. Ann. Genet. 16:285-288, 1973.
46,XX,inv
ins(8)(p22q21),t(1;5;9)(q43;p14q15;p21).
46,XX,inv ins(8)(pter to p22::q21 to p22::q21 to
qter),t(1;5;9)(1pter to 1q43::5q15 to 5qter;9pter
to 9p21::5p14 to 5q15::1q44 to 1qter;9qter to
9p21::5p14 to 5pter).

Same entry as in 01p330 (Pan et al., 1974).

01q440   Negative band

Dewald, G. W., Spurbeck, J. and Gordon, H.:
Automated videodensitometric analysis of autosomal translocations. Amer. J. Hum. Genet.
26:26A, 1974.
Family A in this report.

46,XX and
XY,t(1;9)(q44;p11)?der(9)t(1;9)(q44;p11).

Kreiger, D., Palmer, C. and Biegel, A.: Human
autosomal deletion mapping and HL-A. Humangenetik 23:159-160, 1974.
46,XY,t(1;9)(q44;q11).

Laurent, C., Bovier-Lapierre, M. and Dutrillaux,
B.: Partial trisomy 10 due to hereditary translocation t(1;10)(q44;q22). Humangenetik 18:321-
327, 1973.
46,XX,t(1;10)(q44;q22).
46,XX and XY,der(1)der(10)t(1;10)[q44;q22)mat.
46,XX,-1,+der(1)t(1;10)(q44;q22)mat.
46,XX,-1,+der(1)t(1;10)(1pter to 1q44::10q22 to
10qter)mat.

Steffensen, D. M.: Rotterdam Conference, 1974.
t(1;4)(q44;q25).

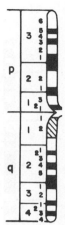

020000

Breg, W. R., Miller, D. A., Allderdice, P. W. and
Miller, O. J.: Identification of translocation
chromosomes by quinacrine fluorescence. Amer. J.
Dis. Child. 123:561-564, 1972.
Patient No. 3 in this report.
46,XX,t(2p6q)t(2q6p).

Deryagin, G. V., Badaev, N. S., Iordamsky, A. B.
and Podugolnikova, O. A.: A study of the spira-
lization dynamics in normal and inverted human
chromosome No. 2. Tsitologiia 16:621-625, 1974.

Jacobs, P. A., Buckton, K. E., Cunningham, C. and
Newton, M. S.: An analysis of the break points
of structural rearrangements in man. J. Med.
Genet. 11:50-64, 1974.
M. R. C. Registry No. K128-227-68 in this report.
46,XX,t(2p7q)t(2q7p).

Merz, T., El-Mahdi, A. M. and Prempree, T.:
Unusual chromosomes and malignant disease.
Lancet 1:337-339, 1968.
One abnormally long chromosome was found in the
karyotypes of individuals with family history of
tumors.

02p000

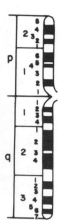

Bender, K., Reinwein, H., Gorman, L. Z. and Wolf, U.: 2-C translocation in father and daughter: 46,XY,t(2p-;Cp+) and 46,XX,Cp+. Humangenetik 8:94-104, 1969.
46,XY,t(2p-;Cp+).
46,XX,-C,+der(C)t(2p-;Cp+)pat.

Same entry as in 0Yq100 (Caspersson et al., 1971).

Chen, A. T. L., Sergovich, F. R., McKim, J. S., Barr, M. L. and Gruber, D.: Chromosome studies in full-term low-birth-weight, mentally retarded patients. J. Pediat. 76:393-398, 1970.
Patient W. M. in this report.
46,XX,inv(2)(pq).

Clark, C.: Balanced autosomal translocation t(2p-;Dq+) in a family. Newport Beach, Calif., Birth Defects Conf., National Foundation - March of Dimes, p. 112, June 16-21, 1974.
46,XY,t(2p-;Dq+).
46,XX,der(2)der(D)t(2p-;Dq+)pat.

de Grouchy, J.: A complex familial chromosome translocation. Amer. J. Hum. Genet. 17:501-509, 1965.
A translocation with one of the B(4-5) group chromosomes has been reported here.

de Grouchy, J., Aussannaire, M., Brissaud, H. E. and Lamy, M.: Aneusomie de Recombinaison: Three further examples. Amer. J. Hum. Genet. 18:467-484, 1966.
Case 2 in this report.
46,XX,t(2;B)(p;p1).
46,XX and XY,der(2),der(B),t(2;B)(p;p1)mat.
Case 3 in this report.
46,XX,inv(2)(pg).

Fitzgerald, M. G.: Complex five-break rearrangement. Clin. Genet. 5:62-67, 1974.
46,XY,t(2p-;3q+),ins(2q+;3p-)nomp.   (Not maternally or paternally inherited).
Banding studies on the patient (R.C.H. 208) showed a unique combination of reciprocal trans-

location and insertion involving chromosomes 2
and 3.

Handmaker, S. D., Hall, B. D. and Conte, F. A.:
A new recognizable syndrome associated with a
chromosomal abnormality. Newport Beach, Calif.,
Birth Defects Conf., National Foundation - March
of Dimes, p. 84, June 16-21, 1974.
46,XX,2p-,4p-,7q+,8q+.
46,XX,der(2p-)der(4p-)der(7q+)der(8q+)mat.

Hulten, M., Lindsten, J., Ming Pen-Ming, L.,
Fraccaro, M., Mannini, A., Tiepolo, L., Robson,
E. B., Heiken, A. and Tillinger, K. G.: Possible
localization of the genes for the Kidd blood
group on an autosome involved in a reciprocal
translocation. Nature 211:1067-1068, 1966.
46,XY,t(2p-;Cp or q+).
46,XX and XY,der(2)der(C)t(2p-;Cp or q+)pat.

Lee, C. S. N., Bowen, P., Rosenblum, H. and
Linasao, L.: Familial chromosome 2/3 translocation ascertained through an infant with multiple
malformations. New Eng. J. Med. 271:12-16, 1964.
46,XX,t(2p-;3q+).
46,XX,-3,+der(3)t(2p-;3q+)mat.

Ruzicska, P. and Czeizel, A.: Cytogenetic
studies on mid trimester abortuses. Humangenetik
10:273-297, 1970.
Case No. 7-66 in this report.
46,XX,2p-q-.

Shokeir, M. H. K., Ying, K. L. and Pabello, P.:
Deletion of the long arm of chromosome No. 7:
Tentative assignment of the Kidd (Jk) locus.
Clin. Genet. 4:360-368, 1973.
46,XX,t(2;7)(p;pq).

Singh, R. P., Jaco, N. T. and Vigna, V.: Pierre
Robin syndrome in siblings. Amer. J. Dis. Child.
120:560-561, 1970.
46,XY,inv(2)(pq).
46,XY,der(2)inv(2)(pq)pat.

Summitt, R. L.: Familial 2/3 translocation.
Amer. J. Hum. Genet. 18:172-186, 1966.
46,XY,t(2p-;3p+).

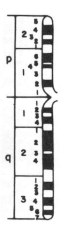

46,XX,der(2)der(3)t(2p-;3p+)mat and pat.
46,XX,-3,+der(3)t(2p-;3p+)mat.
Propositus mi in this report.
46,XY,-3,+der(3)t(2p-;3p+)mat.

Same entry as in 0Y0000 (van den Berghe et al., 1965).

Weitkamp, L. R., Janzen, M. K., Guttormsen, S. A. and Gershowitz, H.: Inherited pericentric inversion of chromosome number two: A linkage study. Ann. Hum. Genet. 33:53-59, 1969.
46,XX and XY,inv(2)(pq).

Wikramanayake, E., Renwick, J. H. and Ferguson-Smith, M. A.: Chromosomal heteromorphisms in the assignment of loci to particular autosomes: A study of four pedigrees. Ann. Genet. 14:245-256, 1971.
Family V21AN in this report.
46,XX and XY,inv(2)(pq).
46,XX and XY,der(2)inv(2)(pq)mat and pat.
A pericentric inversion has been reported here. Since banding techniques were not used, break points cannot be identified.

02p100

Breg, W. R., Miller, D. A., Allderdice, P. W. and Miller, O. J.: Identification of translocation chromosomes by quinacrine fluorescence. Amer. J. Dis. Child. 123:561-564, 1972.
Patient No. 1 in this report.
46,XX,t(2;11)(p1;p1).

Dallapiccola, B.: Familial translocation t(2p-;17p+). Ann. Genet. 14:153-155, 1971.
46,XY,t(2;17)(p1;p1).
46,XX and XY,der(2)der(17)t(2;17)(p1;p1)pat.

Dodson, W. E., Museles, M., Kennedy, J. L. and Al-Aish, M. S.: Acrocephalosyndactyly associated with a chromosomal translocation. Amer. J. Dis. Child. 120:360-362, 1970.
46,XX,t(2;11 or 12)(p1;q2).

Lundsten, C., Vestermark, S. and Philip, J.: A familial, balanced 2/5 translocation associated

with trisomy 21 in one individual. Hum. Hered.
24:88-99, 1974.
46,XX and XY,t(2;5)(p11 or p13;q33 or q35).
46,XX and XY,der(2)der(5)t(2;5)(p11 or p13;q33 or
q35)mat and pat.
47,XY,+21,der(2)der(5)t(2;5)(p11 or p13;q33 or
q35)mat.

Miller, J. R., Dill, F. J., Corey, M. J. and
Rigg, J. M.: A rare translocation [47,XY,t(2p-
;21q+),21+] associated with Down's syndrome. J.
Med. Genet. 7:389-393, 1970.
46,XX,t(2;21)(p1;q2).
46,XX,der(2)der(21)t(2;21)(p1;q2)mat.
47,XY,der(2)der(21)t(2;21)(p1;q2)mat,+21.

Schmid, W. and Hatfield, D.: Normal karyotype/
translocation mosaic. Cytogenetics 1:210-216,
1962.
46,XX/46,XX,tan(2;13, 14 or 15)(p1;q34,q32, or
q26).

Same entry as in 0Yp110 (van den Berghe, Fryns
and David, 1973).

02p110   Negative band

Creasy, M. R. and Crolla, J. A.: Prenatal morta-
lity of trisomy 21 (Down's syndrome). Lancet
1:473-474, 1974.
An abortus was found to have mosaicism with the
cell lines:
46,XY,-2,-21,+t(2p21q),+t(2q21q)/47,XY,+21.
"This was a mosaic with a primary 21-trisomic
cell-line and a cell-line with one normal chromosome 21 and two recombinant chromosomes, one
consisting of the long arms of a 21 and the long
arms of a number 2 and the other composed of the
long arms of a 21 translocated on to the short
arms of the 2. . ."

Jacobs, P. A., Melville, M., Ratcliffe, S., Keay,
A. J. and Syme, J.: A cytogenetic survey of
11,680 newborn infants. Ann. Hum. Genet. 37:359-
376, 1974.
M. R. C. Registry No. 161-72 in this report.
46,XX,inv(2)(p11q13).
46,XX,inv(2)(pter to p11::q13 to p11::q13 to

qter).

02p130   Negative band

Therkelsen, A. J., Hulten, M., Jonasson, J., Lindsten, J., Christensen, N. C. and Iversen, T.: Presumptive direct insertion within chromosome 2 in man. Ann. Hum. Genet. 36:367-373, 1973.
46,XY,ins(2)(q34p13p24).
46,XX and XY,rec(2)dup p,ins(2)(q34p13p24).
Recombinant and inverted insertions have been found in this kindred.

02p200

de Grouchy, J.:   A complex familial chromosome translocation.   Amer. J. Hum. Genet. 17:501-509, 1965.
46,XX and XY,t(2;4 or 5)(p2q1).

02p210   Negative band

Lozzio, C. B. and Klepper, M. B.: Chromosome aberrations identified by the new banding techniques. Amer. J. Hum. Genet. 26:55A, 1974.
t(2;4)(p21;q35)mat.
This familial reciprocal translocation was reported here.

02p230   Negative band

Ferguson-Smith, M. A., Newman, B. F., Ellis, P. M., Thomson, D. M. G. and Riley, I. D.: Assignment by deletion of human red cell acid phosphatase gene locus to the short arm of chromosome 2. Nature (New Biol.) 243:271-274, 1973.
Family BE in this report.
46,XX,t(2;5)(p23;q31)
46,XX,t(2;5)(2qter to 2p23::5q31 to 5qter;5pter to 5q31::2p23 to 2pter).
46,XX and 46,XY,der(2)der(5)t(2;5)(p23;q31)mat.
46,XY,-2,+der(2)t(2;5)(p23;q31)mat.
46,XY,-2,+der(2)t(2;5)(2qter to 2p23::5q31 to 5qter)mat.

02p240   Positive band

Same entry as in 02p130 (Therkelsen et al, 1973).

02p250   Negative band

Same entry as in 01q320 (Alfi, 1973).

Same entry as in 01q320 (Sanger, Alfi and Donnell, 1974).

Subrt, I., Kozak, J. and Hnikova, O.: Microden-
sitometric identification of the pericentric
inversion of chromosome No. 2 and of duplication
of the short arm of chromosome No. 7 in a reexa-
mined case. Hum. Hered. 23:331-337, 1973.
46,XX,inv(2)(p25q13),dup(7)(p14p13 or p13p14).
46,XX,inv(2)(pter to p25::q13 to p25::q13 to
qter),dup(7)(pter to p14::p13 to qter) or du-
p(7)(pter to p13::p14 to qter).

02q000

Bijlsma, J. B., de France, H., Bleeker-Wogema-
kers, E. M. and Wijffels, J. C. H. M.: Duplication deficiency syndrome in familial translocation (2q-;5p+). Humangenetik 12:110-122, 1971.
46,XY,t(2q-;5p+).
46,XX and XY,der(2)der(5)t(2q-;5p+)pat.
Propositus D. W. in this report.
46,XX,-5,+der(5)t(2q-;5p+)mat.
Chromosome identification by autoradiography.

Buckton, K. E.: The identification of whole
chromosomes or parts of chromosomes by the new
banding techniques. Nobel Symposium 23:196-200,
1972.
46,XX,t(2q-;10q+).

Buhler, E. M., Luchsinger, U., Buhler, U. K.,
Mehes, K. and Stalder, G. R.: Non-condensation
of one segment of a chromosome No. 2 in a male
with an otherwise normal karyotype (and severe
hypospadias). Humangenetik 9:97-104, 1970.
A non-condensed (gap-like) region near the
centromere was found.

Daniel, W. L.: A genetic and biochemical investigation of primary microcephaly. Amer. J. Ment.
Defic. 75:653-662, 1971.
46,XX,t(2;C)(q;q).
46,XX,-2,+der(2)t(2;C)(q;q)mat.

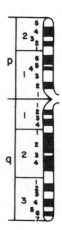

46,XX,-2,+der(2)t(2;C)(2pter to 2q::Cq to Cqter)mat.

Davison, B. C. C., Bedford, J. and Dunn, W.: t(2q-;Dq+) in a mentally retarded female child. J. Med. Genet. 7:81-82, 1970.
46,XX,t(2q-;Dq+).

Same entry as in 02p000 (de Grouchy et al., 1966, case 3).

Ferguson-Smith, M. A.: Inherited constriction fragility of chromosome 2. Ann. Genet. 16:29-34, 1973.
2qh is reported in three generations in a family.

Same entry as in 02p000 (Fitzgerald, 1974).

Genest, P., Lachance, R., Poty, J. and Jacob, D.: Autosomal translocation in a mentally retarded male child with 46,XY,t(2q-;13q+) complement: case report and review. J. Med. Genet. 8:504-508, 1971.
46,XY,t(2q-;13q+).

German, J.: Studying human chromosomes today. Amer. Sci. 58:182-201, 1970.
46,XY,t(2;4)(q;q).
46,XY,t(2;4)(2pter to 2q::4q to 4qter;4pter to 4q::2q to 2qter).

Masterson, J., Law, E., MacDonald, A. and Donovan, D.: Congenital abnormalities in a child with presumptive karyotype 46,XX,t(2q-;17q+). Irish J. Med. Sci. 3:1-4, 1970.
46,XX,t(2q-;17q+).

Neu, R. L. and Gardner, L. I.: Three families with abnormal inherited chromosomes: 2q+mat,t(Cp+;13q-)mat and t(3?-;5q+)pat. Ann. Genet. 15:19-23, 1972.
46,XX,2q+.
46,XY,der(2q+)mat.
Case No. 1 in this report.
46,XX,der(2q+)mat.

Reisman, L. E. and Kasahara, S.: An unusual chromosome abnormality 2/D translocation. Amer.

J. Dis. Child. 115:625-628, 1968.
46,XX,t(2q-;14q+).
Chromosome identification by autoradiography.

Reiss, J. A., Wyandt, H. E., Magenis, R. E.,
Lovrien, E. W. and Hecht, F.: Mosaicism with
translocation: autoradiographic and fluorescent
studies of an inherited reciprocal translocation
t(2q+;14q-). J. Med. Genet. 9:280-286, 1972.
46,XY,t(2q+;14q-).
46,XY,t(2;14)(2pter to 2q::14q to 14qter;14pter
to 14q::2q to 2qter).
46,XY,der(2)der(14)t(2q+;14q-)mat/
47,XY,der(2)der(14)t(2q+;14q-)mat,+
der(14)t(2;14)mat.

Robson, E. B., Polani, P. E., Dart, S. J.,
Jacobs, P. A. and Renwick, J. H.: Probable
assignment of the alpha locus of haptoglobin to
chromosome 16 in man. Nature 223:1163-1165,
1969.
46,XY,t(2q-;16q+).
46,XX and XY,der(2)der(16)t(2q-;16q+)mat and pat.

Same entry as in 02p000 (Ruzicska and Czeizel,
1970).

van den Berghe, H.: Personal Communication,
1974.
46,XX and XY,2qh.
Two boys presented with an apparently identical
and lethal central nervous system disorder (dead
at approximately nine months). The surviving
sister is phenotypically normal. No 2qh was
found in the parents.

Wahrman, J., Goitein, R., Richler, C., Goldman,
B., Akstein, E. and Chaki, R.: The mongoloid
phenotype is due to triplication of the distal
pale G-band of chromosome 21. Leiden Chr. Conf.
Proc.:87, 1974.
46,XX,t(2q-;21q+).
46,XY,der(2)t(2q-;21q+).
Partial trisomy for 21q. The authors hypothesize
that the distal pale G band region of the long
arm is responsible for Down syndrome phenotype.

Same entry as in 02p000 (Weitkamp et al., 1969).

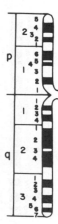

Same entry as in 02p000 (Wikramanayake, Renwick and Ferguson-Smith, 1971).

Wurster, D. H., Hoefnagel, D., Benirschke, K. and Allen, F. H.: Placental chorangiomata and mental deficiency in a child with 2-15 translocation: 46,XX,t(2q-;15q+). Cytogenetics 8:389-399, 1969.
46,XX,t(2q-;15q+).
Chromosome identification by autoradiography.

02q100

Same entry as in 01p300 (Nuzzo et al., 1973).

02q110   Negative band

Jacobs, P. A., Buckton, K. E., Cunningham, C. and Newton, M. S.: An analysis of the break points of structural rearrangements in man. J. Med. Genet. 11:50-64, 1974.
M. R. C. Registry No. K210-190-72 in this report.
46,XX,t(2;10)(q11;q22).

Worton, R. G.: Personal Communication, 1973.
46,XY,t(2;8)(q11;q24).
Mutant Cell Repository No. GM-327.

02q120   Positive band

Leisti, J.: Structural variation in human mitotic chromosomes. Ann. Acad. Sci. fenn. (Med.) Series A, IV, Biologica 179:1-69, 1971.
Case No. 1 in this report.
46,XX,2qh.

Lejeune, J., Dutrillaux, B., Lafourcade, J., Berger, R., Abonyi, D. and Rethore, M. O.: Endoreduplication selective du bras long du chromosome 2 chez une femme et sa fille. C. R. Acad. Sci. Series D 266:24-26, 1968.

Nielsen, J.: Structural aberration in chromosome No. 2. Humangenetik 19:281-284, 1973.
A gap was found at approximately 2q12 in two males with no effect on the phenotype.

02q130   Negative band

Same entry as in 01q320 (Desroches, Bradshaw and Jones, 1973).

Same entry as in 01q320 (Francke, 1974).

German, J. and Chaganti, R. S. K.: Mapping human autosomes: Assignment of the MN locus to a specific segment in the long arm of chromosome No. 2. Science 182:1261-1262, 1973.
46,XY,t(2;4)(q13q21;q31).
46,XY,t(2;4)(2pter to 2q13::4q31 to 4qter;4pter to 4q31::2q21 to 2qter).
A deletion of the band region 2q14 has been hypothesized.

Same entry as in 02p110 (Jacobs et al., 1974).

Kreiger, D., Palmer, C. and Biegel, A.: Human autosomal deletion mapping and EL-A. Humangenetik 23:159-160, 1974.
46,XY,t(2;6)(q13;p23).

Same entry as in 02p250 (Subrt, Kozak and Hnikova, 1973).

02q140   Positive band

Same entry as in 02q130 (German and Chaganti, 1973).

02q200

Lisco, E. and Lisco, H.: A case of a balanced 2/D translocation. Ann. Genet. 10:42, 1967.
46,XX,tan(2;13, 14 or 15)(q2;q3,q3 or q2).

02q210   Negative band

Same entry as in 02q130 (German and Chaganti, 1973).

Weitkamp, L. R.: Rotterdam Conference, 1974.
46,XX and XY,t(2;10)(q21;?).

02q230   Negative band

Jacobs, P. A., Buckton, K. E., Cunningham, C. and Newton, M. S.: An analysis of the break points

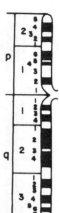

of structural rearrangements in man. J. Med. Genet. 11:50-64, 1974.
M. R. C. Registry No. 119-109-71 in this report.
46,XY,t(2;15)(q23;q21).

02q300

Falk, R. E., Carrel, R. E., Valente, M., Crandall, B. F. and Sparkes, R. S.: Partial trisomy of chromosome 11: A case report. Amer. J. Ment. Defic. 77:383-388, 1973.
46,XY,t(2;11)(q3;p1).
Case RQ 052561 in this report.
46,XY,-2,+der(2)t(2;11)(q3;p1)pat.
46,XY,-2,+der(2)t(2;11)(2pter to 2q3::11p1 to 11pter)pat.
See Francke (1972) in entry 02q300.

Francke, U.: Quinacrine mustard fluorescence of human chromosomes: characterization of unusual translocations. Amer. J. Hum. Genet. 24:189-213, 1972.
46,XY,t(2;11)(q3;p1).
Case No. 7: RQ 052561 in this report.
46,XY,-2,+der(2)t(2;11)(q3;p1)pat.
46,XY,-2,+der(2)t(2;11)(2pter to 2q3::11p1 to 11pter)pat.

Grosse, K. P. and Schwanitz, G.: Diagnostik und genetische Beratung bei reziproken chromosomen-translokationen dargestellt am Beispiel einer familiaren A/E translokation. Mschr. Kinderheilk. 121:108-113, 1973.
46,XX,t(2;18)(q3;q2).
46,XY,t(2;18)(2pter to 2q3::18q2 to 18qter;18pter to 18q2::2q3 to 2qter).
46,XX,der(2)der(18)t(2;18)(q3q2)pat.
46,XX,-2,+der(2)t(2;18)(q3;q2)mat.
46,XX,-2,+der(2)t(2;18)(2pter to 2q3::18q2 to 18qter)mat.

Same entry as in 22q100 (Hayata, Kakati and Sandberg, 1973).

Mercer, R. D. and Darajian, G.: Presumed translocation of chromosome number 2 and one of the D group. Cleveland Clin. Quart. 30:225-232, 1963.
45,XY,t(2;D)(q3;q1).

45,XY,t(2;D)(2pter to 2q3::Dq1 to Dqter).

Shapiro, L. R. and Warburton, D.: Interstitial translocations in man. Lancet 2:712-713, 1972.
46,XX,t(2;12)(q3;q1).
46,XX,t(2;12)(2pter to 2q3?;12pter to 12q1::2q3 to 2qter?::12q1 to 12qter).
46,XX and XY,-12,+der(12)t(2;12)(q3;q1)mat.
46,XX and XY,-12,+der(12)t(2;12)(12pter to 12q1::2q3 to 2qter?::12q1 to 12qter)mat.

02q310   Negative band

Friedrich, U. and Nielsen, J.: Autosomal reci-procal translocations in newborn children and their relatives. Humangenetik 21:133-144, 1974. Proband No. 4838 in this report.
46,XX,t(2;17)(q31;q25).
46,XX,t(2;17)(2pter to 2q31::17q25 to 17qter;17p-ter to 17q25::2q31 to 2qter).

02q320   Positive band

Forabosco, A., Dutrillaux, B., Toni, G., Tam-borino, G. and Cavazzuti, G.: Familial balanced translocation t(2;13)(q32;q33) and partial trisomy 2q. Ann. Genet. 16:255-258, 1973.
46,XX,t(2;13)(q32;q33).
46,XX,t(2;13)(2pter to 2q32;13pter to 13q33::2q32 to 2qter).
46,XX,-13,+der(13)t(2;13)(q32;q33)mat.
46,XX,-13,+der(13)t(2;13)(13pter to 13q33::2q32 to 2qter)mat.

02q330   Negative band

Rosenthal, I. M., Beligere, N., Thompson, F., Pruzansky, S. and Reinglass, H.: Trisomy of the distal portion of the long arm of chromosome 2, a new familial syndrome associated with mental retardation and a characteristic facies. Amer. J. Hum. Genet. 26:73A, 1974.
46,XX,t(2;9)(q33;p24).
46,XX,t(2;9)(2pter to 2q33;9qter to 9p24::2q33 to 2qter).
46,XX,der(2)der(9)t(2;9)(q33;p24)mat.
46,XY,-9,+der(9)t(2;9)(q33;p24)mat.
46,XY,-9,+der(9)t(2;9)(9qter to 9p24::2q33 to

2qter).
The partial trisomy of 2q distal region was found in five individuals in this family.

02q340   Positive band
Same entry as in 02p130 (Therkelsen et al., 1973).

02q370   Negative band

Same entry as in 01p210 (Brown and Shows, 1974).

Same entry as in 01p210 (Shows and Brown, 1974).

030000

Craig-Holmes, A. P., Moore, F. B. and Shaw, M. W.:   Polymorphism of human C-band heterochromatin. I. Frequency of variants. Amer. J. Hum. Genet. 25:181-192, 1973.

Falek, A., Schmidt, R. and Jervis, G. A.: Familial de Lange syndrome with chromosome abnormalities. Pediatrics 37:92-101, 1966.

Gropp, A., Marsch, W. and Brodehl, J.: Structural (translocation) heterozygosity over three subsequent generations in man. Nature 207:374-376, 1965.
46,XX and XY,t(3;C).

Leisti, J.:   Structural variation in human mitotic chromosomes.   Ann. Acad. Sci. fenn. (Med.) Series A, IV, Biologica 179:1-69, 1971.
Case No. 18 in this report.
46,XY,t(3-;16q+).

McHugh, J., Wright, T. and Cooke, P.: A family showing transmission of a translocation t(3p or q-;Cq+).   J. Med. Genet. 8:509-512, 1971.
46,XY,t(3p or q-;Cq+).
46,XY,der(3)der(C)t(3p or q-;Cq+)pat.
46,XX,-C,+der(C)t(3p or q-;Cq+)pat.

Same entry as in 0Xp200 (Mukerjee and Burdette, 1966).

Neu, R. L. and Gardner, L. I.:   Three families

with abnormal chromosomes: 2q+mat,t(Cp+;13q-)mat
and t(3?-;5q+)pat.   Ann. Genet. 15:19-23, 1972.
46,XY,t(3?-;5q+).
46,XX,der(3)der(5)t(3?-;5q+)pat.
Case No. 3 in this report.
46,XY,der(3)der(5)t(3?-;5q+)pat.

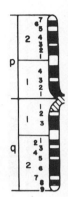

Soukup, S. W., Passarge, E., Becroft, D. M. O.,
Shaw, R. L. and Young, L. G.: Familial translocation (3?-;G?q+) and nondisjunction of chromosome in group G in two unrelated families.
Cytogenetics 8:315-325, 1969.
Partial pedigree of Case No. 1 in this report.
46,XX,t(3?-;G?q+).
46,XX and XY,der(3)der(G)t(3?-;G?q+)mat and pat.
Case No. 1 in this report.
47,XY,der(3)der(G)t(3?-;G?q+)pat,+21.
Partial pedigree of Case No. 2 in this report.
46,XX,t(3?-;G?q+).
46,XY,der(3)der(G)t(3?-;G?q+)mat.
47,XY,der(3)der(G)t(3?-;G?q+)mat,+21.

Walzer, S., Favara, B., Ming, P. L. and Gerald,
P. S.: A new translocation syndrome (3/B). New
Eng. J. Med. 275:290-298, 1966.
46,XY,t(3;B)(p or q,p).

03p000

Same entry as in 01p000 (Buckton, 1972).

Cohen, M. M. and Davidson, R. G.: An inherited
pericentric chromosomal inversion (46,inv3[p-q+])
associated with skeletal anomalies. J. Pediat.
79:456-462, 1971.
46,XX,inv(3)(pq).
46,XX,der(3)inv(3)(pq)mat.

del Amo, A., Bueno, M., Gullon, A., Martinez-
lage, M. and Argemt, J.: 46,XY,t(3p-;9q+) with
mental deficiency and congenital malformations.
Genetica Iberia 23:127-143, 1971.
Case MA 261066 in this report.
46,XY,t(3p-;9q+).

del Amo, A. and Gullon, A.: Familial translocation t(3p+;8q-) studied by banding with Giemsa
staining. Humangenetik 15:14-19, 1972.

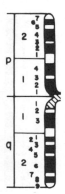

46,XX,t(3p+;8q-).
46,XX and XY,der(3)der(8)t(3p+;8q-)mat.
Case MA 291033 in this report.
46,XY,der(3)der(8)t(3p+;8q-).

Same entry as in 02p000 (Fitzgerald, 1974).

Lejeune, J.:   Scientific impact of the study of
fine   structure   of   chromatids. Nobel Symposium
23:16-24, 1973.
46,X?,ins(7;3)(q3;p14p25)ins(7q+;3p-).

Picciano,   D. J.,   Berlin,   C. M.,   Davenport, S. L.
H.   and Jacobson, C. B.:   Human ring chromosomes:
a   report of five cases.   Ann. Genet. 15:241-247,
1972.
Case No. 1 in this report.
46,XY/46,XY,r(3).

Subrt, I. and Prchlikova, H.:   Double chromosomal
aberration.   Trisomy G and the balanced translocation   t(3p-;17q+).   Humangenetik 8:111-114,
1969.
46,XY,t(3p-;17q+).
46,XX,der(3)der(17)t(3p-;17q+)pat.
Case TZ 111068 in this report.
47,XY,+21,der(3)der(17)t(3p-;17q+).
See entry 03p140 (Subrt, 1974).

Same entry as in 02p000 (Summitt, 1966).

03p100

Breg, W. R., Miller, D. A., Allderdice, P. W. and
Miller,   O.   J.:   Identification of translocation
chromosomes   by quinacrine fluorescence. Amer. J.
Dis. Child. 123:561-564, 1972.
Patient No. 2 in this report.
46,XX,t(3;18)(p1;q1).

03p110   Variable band

Jacobs, P. A., Buckton, K. E., Cunningham, C. and
Newton,   M.   S.:   An analysis of the break points
of   structural   rearrangements   in   man.   J. Med.
Genet. 11:50-64, 1974.
M. R. C. Registry No. K87-200-70 in this report.
46,XY,t(3;19)(p11;p13).

03p130   Negative band

Soudek, D., O'Shaughnessy, S., Laraya, P. and McCreary, B. D.: Pericentric inversion of "fluorescent" segment in chromosome No. 3. Humangenetik 22:343-346, 1974.
Family L in this report.
46,XY,inv(3)(p13q12).
46,XY,inv(3)(pter to p13::q12 to p13::q12 to qter).
46,XX and XY,der(3)inv(3)(p13q12)pat.
Three unrelated cases of pericentric inversion were identified. Two other cases are identified as A.C. and L.F. in this report. Still more data than that reported earlier (Soudek et al., 1974) are reported on this familial inversion in their abstract report.

03p140   Positive band

Betz, A., Trudeau, C. and de Grouchy, J.: Heterozygosity and homozygosity for a pericentric inversion of the human 3 chromosome. Ann. Genet. 17:77-80, 1974.
46,XX and XY,inv(3)(p14q24).
46,XX and XY,inv(3)(pter to p14::q24 to p14::q24 to qter).
46,XX and XY,der(3)inv(3)(p14q24)mat and pat.
46,XX,der(3)inv(3)(p14q24)mat,der(3)inv(3)(p14q24) pat.

Jacobs, P. A., Buckton, K. E., Cunningham, C. and Newton, M. S.: An analysis of the break points in structural rearrangements in man. J. Med. Genet. 11:50-64, 1974.
M. R. C. Registry No. K66-201-69 in this report.
46,XY,inv(3)(p14q27).
46,XY,inv(3)(pter to p14::q27 to p14::q27 to qter).

Subrt, I.: Verification of the previously reported t(3p-;17q+) by G banding. Humangenetik 23:233-234, 1974.
46,XY,t(3;17)(p14;q23).
46,XY,t(3;17)(3qter to 3p14::17q23 to 17qter;17pter to 17q23::3p14 to 3pter).
46,XX,der(3)der(17)t(3;17)(p14;q23)pat.
47,XY,+21,der(3)der(17)t(3;17)(p14;q23)pat.

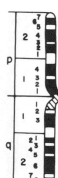

See entry 03p000 (Subrt and Prchlikova, 1969).

03p200

Butler, L. J., Hall, M. E. and Wharton, B. A.: A retarded child with a 46XX,3p-q+ chromosome karyotype. J. Ment. Defic. Res. 18:41-49, 1974.
46,XX,inv(3)(p2q1).
46,XX,inv(3)(pter to p2::q1 to p2::q1 to qter).

Same entry as in 01p320 (Jacobs et al., 1974).

Patau, K., Opitz, J. M. and Dewey, W. L.: A multiple congential anomaly in man presumably caused by a minute deletion in chromosome No. 3. Science 146:429, 1964.
46,XY,t(3;D or G)(p2;p1).
46,XY,der(3)der(D or G)t(3;D or G)(p2;p1)pat.
46,XY,-3,+der(3)t(3;D or G)(p2;p1)pat.
46,XY,-3,+der(3)t(3;D or G)(3qter to 3p2::D or Gp1 to D or Gpter)pat.

03p210   Negative band

Rethore, M. O., Lejeune, J., Carpentier, S., Prieur, M., Dutrillaux, B., Seringe, P., Rossier, A. and Job, J. C.:   Trisomy for the distal portion of the short arm of chromosome No. 3 in three sibs. First instance of chromosomal insertion: Ins(7;3)(q31;p21p26). Ann. Genet. 15:159-165, 1972.
46,XX,?inv ins(7;3)(q31;p21p26).
46,XX,?inv ins(7;3)(7pter to 7q31::3p21 to 3p26::7q31 to 7qter;3pter to 3p26::3p21 to 3qter).
46,XY,-7,+der(7)?inv ins(7;3)(q31;p21p26)mat.
46,XY,-7,+der(7)?inv ins(7;3)(7pter to 7q31::3p21 to 3p26::7q31 to 7qter)mat.

03p250   Negative band

Allderdice, P. W.: Identification of the location of a cross-over in a pericentric inversion heterozygote which resulted in a duplication deficient chromosome 3.   Amer. J. Hum. Genet. 25:11a, 1973, and personal communication, 1973.
46,XY,inv(3)(p25q21).
46,XY,inv(3)(pter to p25::q21 to p25::q21 to

qter).
Offspring with duplication-deficiency resulting
from this inversion have also been found.
See also 03p250 (Hirschhorn, Lucas and Wallace,
1973).

Allderdice, P. W.: A large kindred with segregation of pericentric inversion heterozygotes
inv(3)(p25q21) and inv(8)(p23q22). Amer. J. Hum.
Genet. 26:9A, 1974.
The pericentric inversion has been segregating
for at least seven generations in a large
kindred. Two individuals with a rec(3)dup-
qinv(3)(p25q21) were found.

Baheux-Morlier, G., Taillemite, J. L. and Roux,
C.: Familial occurrence of a translocation t(3q-
;12q+). Ann. Genet. 16:131-134, 1973.
46,XY,t(3;12)(q1;q2).
46,XX,der(3)der(12)t(3;12)(q1;q2)pat.

Boue, J. and Boue, A.: L'interet en diagnostic
prenatal des techniques nouvelles d'identification chromosomique dans des translocations et une
aneusomie de recombinaison. Nouv. Presse Med.
2:3097-3102, 1973.
Observation No. 2822 in this report.
46,XY,inv(3)(p25q21).
46,XY,inv(3)(pter to p25::q21 to p25::q21 to
qter).
See also 03p250 (Hirschhorn, Lucas and Wallace,
1973).

Hirschhorn, K., Lucas, M. and Wallace, I.:
Precise identification of various chromosomal
abnormalities. Ann. Hum. Genet. 36:375-379,
1973.
Family B(Gc 829) in this report.
46,XY,inv(3)(p25q21).
46,XY,inv(3)(pter to p25::q21 to p25::q21 to
qter).
Two offspring (one fetus) with duplication-
deficiency resulting from this inversion are also
reported.
The preceding three reports of inversion may
concern members of a single large kindred (Allderdice, 1973; Boue and Boue, 1973; Hirschhorn et
al., 1973). Attempts are being made to document

this impression.

03p260   Positive band

Same entry as in 03p210 (Rethore et al., 1972).

03q000

Same entry as in 01p000 (Buckton, 1972).

Same entry as in 02p000 (Fitzgerald, 1974).

Same entry as in 02p000 (Lee et al., 1964).

Neu, R. L., Barlow, M. J. and Gardner, L. I.: A case of 46,XY,t(3q-;14q+)mat. Clin. Genet. 4:158-161, 1973.
46,XX,t(3q-;14q+).
46,XY,der(3)der(14)t(3q-;14q+)mat.

03q100

Baheux-Morlier, G., Taillemite, J. L. and Roux, C.: Familial occurrence of a translocation t(3q-;12q+). Ann. Genet. 16:131-134, 1973.
46,XY,t(3;12)(q1;q2).
46,XX,der(3)der(12)t(3;12)q1;q2)pat.

Same entry as in 03p200 (Butler, Hall and Wharton, 1974).

Herrmann, J., Ruffle, T., Meisner, L. F., Viseskul, C. and Gilbert, E. F.: The partial trisomy 3q syndrome. Newport Beach, Calif., Birth Defects Conf., National Foundation - March of Dimes, p. 129, 1974.
46,XX and XY,t(3;12)(q1;q).
46,XY,-12,+der(12)(3;12(q1;q)?.
46,XY,-12,+der(12)t(3;12)(12pter to 12q::3q1 to 3qter)?.

Jacobs, P. A., Buckton, K. E., Cunningham, C. and Newton, M. S.: An analysis of the break points of structural rearrangements in man. J. Med. Genet. 11:50-64, 1974.
M. R. C. Registry No. K83-209-70 in this report.
46,XX,t(3;13)(q12 or 13;q31).

03q110   Variable band

   Uchida, I. A. and Lin, C. C.: Genetic segregation of a fluorescent marker on chromosome No. 3.
   Excerpta Medica, Fourth Int. Cong. Hum. Genet.
   233:180, 1971.
   Segregation of this marker chromosome was studied
   in 20 families.

03q120   Negative band

   Same entry as in 0Xq260 (Pearson, van der Linden
   and Hagemeijer, 1974).

   Same entry as in 03p130 (Soudek et al., 1974).

03q130   Positive band

   Same entry as in 0Xq280 (de la Chapelle and
   Schroder, 1974).

   Same entry as in 0Xq280 (Klinger and de la
   Chapelle, 1974).

03q200

   Altman, A. J., Palmer, C. G. and Baehner, R. L.:
   Juvenile "chronic granulocytic" leukemia: A
   panmyelopathy with prominent monocytic involvement and circulating monocyte colony-forming
   cells. Blood 43:341-350, 1974.
   46,XY,t(3;7)(q2;q2).
   The abnormal translocation was found in three
   cells of a patient with juvenile chronic granulocytic leukemia. All other cells had normal male
   karyotypes.

03q210   Negative band

   Same entry as in 03p250 (Allderdice, 1973).

   Same entry as in 03p250 (Boue and Boue, 1973).

   Same entry as in 03p250 (Hirschhorn, Lucas and
   Wallace, 1973).

   Same entry as in 01p320 (Jacobs et al., 1974).

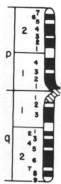

Kreiger, D., Palmer, C. and Biegel, A.: Human autosomal deletion mapping and HL-A. Humangenetik 23:159-160, 1974.
46,XX,t(3;9)(q21;p22).
46,XX,-9,+der(9)t(3;9)(q21;p22)mat.

03q240   Positive band

Same entry as in 03p140 (Betz, Trudeau and de Grouchy, 1974).

03q270   Negative band

Grace, E., Sutherland, G. R. and Bain, A. D.: Familial insertional translocation. Lancet 2:231, 1972.
46,XX,ins(3;7)(q27;q22q32).
46,XX,ins(3;7)(3pter to 3q27::7q22 to 7q32::3q27 to 3qter;7pter to 7q22::7q32 to 7qter).
46,XX,-3,+der(3)ins(3;7)(q27;q22q32)mat.
46,XX,-3,+der(3)ins(3;7)(3pter to 3q27::7q22 to 7q32::3q27 to 3qter)mat.
Also see Grace, E., Sutherland, G. R. and Bain, A. D.: Partial trisomy of 7q resulting from a familial translocation. Ann. Genet. 16:51-54, 1973.

Same entry as in 03p140 (Jacobs et al., 1974).

03q280   Positive band

Friedrich, U. and Nielsen, J.: Autosomal reciprocal translocations in newborn children and their relatives. Humangenetik 21:133-144, 1974.
46,XX,t(3;10)(q28;q22).
46,XX,t(3;10)(3pter to 3q28::10q22 to 10qter;10pter to 10q22::3q28 to 3qter).
46,XY,der(3)der(10)t(3;10)(q28;q22)mat.
Proband No. 9226 in this report.
46,XX,der(3)der(10)t(3;10)(q28;q22)pat.

03q290   Negative band

Jacobs, P. A., Buckton, K. E., Cunningham, C. and Newton, M. S.: An analysis of the break points of structural rearrangements in man. J. Med. Genet. 11:50-64, 1974.
M. R. C. Registry No. K134-14-71 in this report.

46,XY,t(3;20)(q29;p11).

Kreiger, D., Palmer, C. and Biegel, A.: Human autosomal deletion mapping and HL-A. Humangenetik 23:159-160, 1974.
46,XX,t(3;13)(q29;q14).

040000

Carrel, R. E., Sparkes, R. S. and Wright, S. W.: Chromosome survey of moderately to profoundly retarded patients. Amer. J. Ment. Defic. 47:616-622, 1973.
45,XX,-4,-13,+t(4q13q).

04p100

Bobrow, M., Jones, L. F. and Clarke, G.: A complex chromosomal rearrangement with formation of a ring 4. J. Med. Genet. 8:235-239, 1971.
46,XY,r(4)(p1q3),t(4;17 or 18)(q3;p1).
46,XY,r(4)(p1 to q3),t(4;17 or 18)(4qter to 4q3::17 or 18p1 to 17 or 18qter).

Breg, W. R.: 1973.
46,XY,del(4)(p1).
46,XY,del(4)(qter to p1:).
Mutant Cell Repository No. GM-72.

Carrel, R. E., Sparkes, R. S. and Wright, S. W.: Chromosome survey of moderately to profoundly retarded patients. Amer. J. Ment. Defic. 47:616-622, 1973.
46,XY/46,XY,r(4)/46,XY,4q-.

Carter, R., Baker, E. and Hayman, D.: Congenital malformations associated with a ring 4 chromosome. J. Med. Genet. 6:224-227, 1969.
46,XY,r(4).
The ring chromosome was not identified by autoradiography but it was considered to be a No. 4, because the associated congenital abnormalities are similar to those described in cases of deletion of the short arm of chromosome number 4.

Fryns, J. P., Eggermont, E., Verresen, H. and van den Berghe, H.: The 4p- syndrome, with a report of two new cases. Humangenetik 19:99-109,

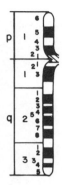

1973.
46,XY,del(4)(p1).
46,XY,del(4)(qter to p1:).
Wolf syndrome. Previous reports are reviewed
here.

Gouw, W. L., Anders, G. J. P. A., ten Kate, L. P.
and de Groot, C. J.: Paternal transmission of a
B/D translocation, t(4p-;14p+ or 15p+), resulting
in a partial 4p trisomy. Humangenetik 16:251-
259, 1972.
46,XY,t(4;14 or 15)(p1;p1).
46,XY,-14 or -15,+der(14 or 15)t(4;14 or
15)(p1;p1)pat.
46,XY,-14 or -15,+der(14 or 15)t(4;14 or 15)(14
or 15qter to 14 or 15p1::4p1 to 4pter)pat.

Guthrie, R. D., Aase, J. M., Asper, A. C. and
Smith, D. W.: The 4p- syndrome. A clinically
recognizable chromosomal deletion syndrome.
Amer. J. Dis. Child. 122:421-425, 1971.

Same entry as in 02p000 (Handmaker, Hall and
Conte, 1974).

Hirschhorn, K., Cooper, H. L. and Firschein, I.
L.: Deletion of short arms of chromosome 4-5 in
a child with defects of midline fusion. Humangenetik 1:479-482, 1965.
46,XY,del(4)(p1).
46,XY,del(4)(qter to p1:).

Jacobs, P. A., Buckton, K. E., Cunningham, C. and
Newton, M. S.: An analysis of the break points
of structural rearrangements in man. J. Med.
Genet. 11:50-64, 1974.
M. R. C. Registry No. K35-116-67 in this report.
46,XY,t(4;18)(p12 or 13 or 14;q2).

Metz, F., Bier, L. and Pfeiffer, R. A.: Partial
trisomy of the short arm of chromosome 4 due to
translocation t(4p-22p+). Humangenetik 18:207-
211, 1973.
46,XY,t(4;22)(p1;p1).
46,XY,t(4;22)(4qter to 4p1::22p1 to 22pter;22qter
to 22p1::4p1 to 4pter).
46,XX and XY,der(4)der(22)t(4;22)(p1;p1)pat.
46,XX,-22,+der(22)t(4;22)(p1;p1)mat.

46,XX,-22,+der(22)t(4;22)(22qter   to 22p1::4p1 to
4pter)mat.

Mikelsaar, A. V. N., Lazjuk, G. J., Lurie, J. W.,
Tuur, S. J., Kyaosaar, M. E., Mikelsaar, R. and
Loolaid, V. E.: A 4p- syndrome. Humangenetik
19:345-347, 1973.
46,XX,del(4)(p1).
46,XX,del(4)(4qter to 4p1:).

Miller, O. J., Breg, W. R., Warburton, D.,
Miller, D. A., de Capoa, A., Allderdice, P. W.,
Davis, J., Klinger, H. P., McGilvray, E. and
Allen, F. H.: Partial deletion of the short arm
of chromosome No. 4 (4p-): Clinical studies in
five unrelated patients. J. Pediat. 77:792-801,
1970.
Patient 4 (KR261252), patient 11 (PM290664),
patient 19 (RF281059), patient 24 (MB201067), and
patient 28 (ME200267) in this report.
46,XX and XY,del(4)(p1).
46,XX and XY,del(4)(qter to p1:).

Miller, D. A., Warburton, D. and Miller, O. J.:
Clustering in deleted short-arm length among 25
cases with a Bp- chromosome. Cytogenetics
8:109-116, 1969.
46,XX and XY,4p-.

Schinzel, A. and Schmid, W.: Partial trisomy for
the short arm of chromosome 4 with translocation
4p-,18q+ in the father. Humangenetik 15:163-171,
1972.
46,XY,t(4p-,18q+).
46,XY,-18,+der(18)t(4p-;18q+)pat,+16q+.
Chromosome identification by autoradiography.

Schmid, W.: The prenatal diagnosis of chromosome
anomalies. Triangle 11:91-102, 1972.
46,XY,t(4;18)(p1;q),16qh+.
46,XY,-18,+der(8)t(4;18)(p1;q)pat,der(16qh+)pat.
46,XY,-18,+der(8)t(4;18)(18pter to 18q::4p1 to
4pter)pat,der(16qh+)pat.

Surana, R. B., Bailey, J. D. and Conen, P. E.: A
ring 4 chromosome in a patient with normal
intelligence and short stature. J. Med. Genet.
8:517-521, 1971.

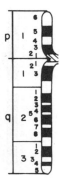

46,XX,r(4)(pq).

Taillemite, J. L., Baheux-Morlier, G., Cathelineau, L. and Roux, C.: Cri du chat syndrome and complex chromosome rearrangement in a dizygotic twin. Ann. Genet. 16:127-130, 1973.
46,XX,5p-,ins(4;13)(p1;q).

Warburton, D. and Miller, O. J.: Dermatoglyphic features of patients with a partial short arm deletion of a B-group chromosome. Ann. Hum. Genet. 31:189-207, 1967.

Wilson, M. G., Towner, J. W., Coffin, G. S. and Forsman, I.: Inherited pericentric inversion of chromosome No. 4. Amer. J. Hum. Genet. 22:679-690, 1970.
46,XX,inv(4)(pq).
46,XX,der(4)inv(4)(pq)mat.

Wilson, M. G., Towner, J. W. and Negus, L. D.: Wolf-Hirschhorn syndrome associated with an unusual abnormality of chromosome No. 4. J. Med. Genet. 7:164-170, 1970.
46,XY,4p+.

Wolf, U., Porsch, R., Baitsch, H. and Reinwein, H.: Deletion on short arms of a B-chromosome without "cri-du-chat" syndrome. Lancet 1:769, 1965.

Wolf, U., Reinwein, H., Porsch, R., Schroter, R. and Baitsch, H.: Defizienz an den kurzen Armen eines chromosoms Nr. 4. Humangenetik 1:397-413, 1965.
46,XX,del(4)(p1).
46,XX,del(4)(qter to p1:).
A portion of the short arm is deleted in this condition which has been called 'Wolf-Hirschhorn' syndrome.

04p110   Variable band

Giovannelli, G., Forabosco, A. and Dutrillaux, B.: Familial translocation t(4;22)(p11;p12) and trisomy 4p in two sibs. Ann. Genet. 17:119-124, 1974.
46,XX,t(4;22)(p11;p12).

Cases 1 and 2 in this report.
46,XX,-22,+der(22)t(4;22)(p11;p12)mat.
46,XX,-22,+der(22)t(4;22)(22qter to 22p12::4p11
to 4pter)mat.

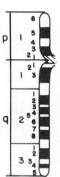

Giovannelli, G., Rossi, L. and Forabosco, A.:
Radiological findings in two sisters with trisomy
of the short arm of chromosome 4. Helv. Paediat.
Acta 28:543-552, 1973.
46,XX,t(4;22)(p11;p12).
Cases 1 and 2 in this report.
46,XX,-22,+der(22)t(4;22)(p11;p12)mat.
46,XX,-22,+der(22)t(4;22)(22qter to 22p12::4p11
to 4pter)mat.

Seabright, M.: Personal Communication, 1974).
46,XY,der(21)t(4;21)(p11;p12).
Mutant Cell Repository No. GM-98.

04p120   Negative band

Lozzio, C. B. and Klepper, M. B.: Chromosome
aberrations identified by the new banding techniques. Amer. J. Hum. Genet. 26:55A, 1974.
inv(4)(p12q34).
This familial inversion is reported here.

04p130   Positive band

Dallapiccola, B., Capra, L., Preto, G., Covic, M.
and Dutrillaux, B.:   Pericentric inversion of
chromosome 4: inv(4)(p13q35) and trisomy 4p by
aneusomie de recombinaison. Ann. Genet. 17:115-
118, 1974.
46,XY,inv(4)(p13q35).
46,XY,inv(4)(pter to p13::q35 to p13::q35 to
qter).
46,XY,der(4)inv(4)(p13q35)pat.
46,XY,rec(4)dup inv(4)(p13q35)pat.

04p140   Negative band

Hecht, F.: Personal Communication, 1974.
46,XY,inv(4)(p14q22).
Mutant Cell Repository No. GM-413.
46,XX,inv(4)(p14;q22).
Mutant Cell Repository No. GM-414.

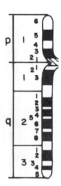

Jacobs, P. A., Buckton, K. E., Cunningham, C. and Newton, M. S.: An analysis of the break points of structural rearrangements in man. J. Med. Genet. 11:50-64, 1974.
M. R. C. Registry No. K192-297-71 in this report.
46,XX,t(4;13)(p14;q14).
M. R. C. Registry No. K57-210-68 in this report.
46,XY,t(4;18)(p14;q11).

Rethore, M. O., Dutrillaux, B., Job, J. C. and Lejeune, J.: Trisomy 4p by aneusomie de recombinaison of an inv(4)(p14q35). Ann. Genet. 17:109-114, 1974.
46,XY,inv(4)(p14q35).
46,XY,inv(4)(pter to p14::q35 to p14::q35 to qter).
46,XY,der(4)inv(4)(p14q35)pat.
46,XY,rec(4)dup p inv(4)(p14q35)pat.

Schwanitz, G. and Grosse, K. P.: Partial trisomy 4p with translocation 4p-,22p+ in the father. Ann. Genet. 16:263-266, 1973.
46,XY,t(14;22)(p14;p11).
46,XY,t(14;22)(4qter to 4p14::22p11 to 22pter;22qter to 22p11::4p14 to 4pter).
46,XX and XY,-22,+der(22)t(4;22)(p14;p11)pat.
46,XX and XY,-22,+der(22)t(4;22)(22qter to 22p11::4p14 to 4pter)pat.

04p150   Positive band

Kreiger, D., Palmer, C. and Biegel, A.: Human autosomal deletion mapping and HL-A. Humangenetik 23:159-160, 1974.
46,XX,del(4)(p15).
46,XX,del(4)(qter to p15:).

04p160   Negative band

Jacobs, P. A., Buckton, K. E., Cunningham, C. and Newton, M. S.: An analysis of the break points of structural rearrangements in man. J. Med. Genet. 11:50-64, 1974.
M. R. C. Registry No. K184-225-71 in this report.
46,XY,t(4;6)(p16;p11).

04p200

Same entry as in 01p000 (Gray et al., 1972).

04q000

Bobrow, M., Jones, L. F. and Clarke, G.: A complex chromosomal rearrangement with formation of a ring 4. J. Med. Genet. 8:235-239, 1971.

Bobrow, M. and Pearson, P. L.: The use of quinacrine fluorescence in the identification of B and E group chromosomes involved in structural abnormalities. J. Med. Genet. 8:240-243, 1971.
45,XX or XY,-4,-18,+t(4;18)(q;p11).
45,XX or XY,-4,-18,+t(4;18)(18qter to 18p11::4q to 4qter).

Buckton, K. E.: The identification of whole chromosomes or parts of chromosomes by the new banding techniques. Nobel Symposium 23:196-200, 1972.
46,XY,t(4q-;9p+).

Same entry as in 04p100 (Carrel, Sparkes and Wright, 1973).

Carrel, R. E., Sparkes, R. S. and Wright, S. W.: Chromosome survey of moderately to profoundly retarded patients. Amer. J. Ment. Defic. 47:616-622, 1973.
46,XY,4q+.

Centerwall, W. R., Thompson, W. P., Allen, I. E. and Fobes, C. D.: The Wolf (4p-) syndrome in other clothes - A case report and an overall review. Amer. J. Hum. Genet. 26:19A, 1974.
46,XX,-4,-22,+t(4q22q1).

Cohen, M. M., Lin, C. C. and Davidson, R. G.: Two B-C translocations specifically identified by 'banding' techniques. J. Med. 3:216-223, 1972.
Patient V. K. in this report.
46,XX,t(4q-;7p+).

Same entry as in 02q000 (German, 1970).

German, J.: Studying human chromosomes today. Amer. Sci. 58:182-201, 1970.
46,XX,4q+.

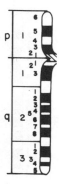

"An extra segment of some chromosome has been translocated to the long arm of a No. 4."

Grotsky, H., Hsu, L. Y. F. and Hirschhorn, K.: A case of cri-du-chat associated with cataracts and transmitted from a mother with 4/5 translocation. J. Med. Genet. 8:369-371, 1971.
46,XX,t(4q+;5p-).
46,XX,-5,+der(5p-)t(4q+;5p-)mat.

Hoehn, H., Sander, C. and Sander, L. Z.: Aneusomie de recombinaison: rearrangement between paternal chromosomes 4 and 18 yielding offspring with features of the 18q- syndrome. Ann. Genet. 14:187-192, 1971.
46,XY,t(4q-;18q+).
46,XY,der(4)der(18)t(4q-;18q+)pat.
Chromosome identification by autoradiography.

Jacobs, P. A., Buckton, K. E., Cunningham, C. and Newton, M. S.: An analysis of the break points of structural rearrangements in man. J. Med. Genet. 11:50-64, 1974.
M. R. C. Registry No. K105-176-69 in this report.
46,XY,t(4;10)(q1 or 21;q22, 23, 24, 25 or 26).
Same patient reported by Newton et al., 1972.

Leisti, J.: Structural variation in human mitotic chromosomes. Ann. Acad. Sci. fenn. (Med.) Series A, IV, Biologica 179:1-69, 1971.
Case 4 in this report.
46,XX,4q-.

Same entry as in 01p000 (Lubs and Lubs, 1974).

Newton, M. S., Cunningham, C., Jacobs, P. A., Price, W. H. and Fraser, I. A.: Chromosome survey of a hospital for the mentally subnormal. Part 2: Autosome abnormalities. Clin. Genet. 3:226-248, 1972.
M. R. C. Registry No. K105-176-69 in this report.
46,XY,t(4q-;10q+).
Same patient reported by Jacobs et al., 1974.

Surana, R. B. and Conen, P. E.: Partial trisomy 4 resulting from a 4/18 reciprocal translocation. Ann. Genet. 15:191-194, 1972.
46,XX,t(4q-;18q+).

46,XX,-18,+der(18)t(4q-;18q+)mat.

Same entry as in 04p100 (Wilson et al., 1970).

04q200

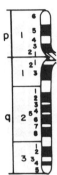

Francke, U.: Quinacrine mustard fluorescence of human chromosomes: characterization of unusual translocations. Amer. J. Hum. Genet. 24:189-213, 1972.
46,XX,t(4;20)(q2;q1).
Case 5: MS 140167 in this report.
46,XY,-20,+der(20)t(4;20)(q2;q1)mat.
46,XY,-20,+der(20)t(4;20)(20pter to 20q1::4q2 to 4qter)mat.

Same entry as in 01p000 (Gray et al., 1972).

Jacobs, P. A., Buckton, K. E., Cunningham, C. and Newton, M. S.: An analysis of the break points of structural rearrangements in man. J. Med. Genet. 11:50-64, 1974.
M. R. C. Registry No. K17-107-65 in this report.
46,XX,t(4;17)(q2;q2).

Schrott, H. G., Sakaguchi, S., Francke, U., Luzzatti, L. and Fialkow, P. J.: Translocation, t(4q-;13q+), in three generations resulting in partial trisomy of the long arm of chromosome 4 in the fourth generation. J. Med. Genet. 11:201-205, 1974.
46,XX,t(4;13)(q26 or q27;q34).
46,XX,t(4;13)(4pter to 4q26 or q27::13q34 to 13qter;13pter to 13q34::4q26 or q27 to 4qter).
46,XX,der(4)der(13)(q26 or q27;q34)mat.
46,XY,-13,+der(13)t(4;13)(q26 or q27;q34)mat.

04q210   Negative band

de la Chapelle, A., Koivisto, M. and Schroder, J.: Segregating reciprocal (4;21)(q21;q21) translocation with proposita trisomic for parts of 4q and 21. J. Med. Genet. 10:384-389, 1973.
46,XY,t(4;21)(q21;q21).
46,XY,t(4;21)(4pter to 4q21::21q21 to 21qter;21pter to 21q21::4q21 to 4qter).
46,XX and XY,der(4)der(21)t(4;21)(q21;q21)pat.
47,XX,+der(21)t(4;21)(q21;q21)mat.

47,XX,+der(21)t(4;21)(21pter to 21q21::4q21 to 4qter)mat.

04q220   Positive band

Same entry as in 04p140 (Hecht, 1974).

04q230   Negative band

Hermann, B., Disteche, C., Ghymers, D. and Frederic, J.: A case of lengthening of a B4 chromosome; Demonstration of an insertion within the long arms [46,XX:ins(4;?)(q23;?)]. Humangenetik 22:255-260, 1974.

04q250   Negative band

Kousseff, B.: Personal Communication, 1974.
46,XX,t(4;11)(q25;q13).
Mutant Cell Repository No. GM-380.

Same entry as in 01q440 (Steffensen, 1974).

04q260   Positive band

Hirschhorn, K., Lucas, M. and Wallace, I.: Precise identification of various chromosomal abnormalities. Ann. Hum. Genet. 36:375-379, 1973.
Family W(Gc 334) in this report.
46,XY,t(4;12)(q26;q12).
46,XY,t(4;12)(4pter to 4q26::12q12 to 12qter;12pter to 12q12::4q26 to 4qter).
46,XY,der(4)der(12)t(4;12)(q26;q12)pat.
46,XX,-4,+der(4)t(4;12)(q26;q12)pat.
46,XX,-4,+der(4)t(4;12)(4pter to 4q26::12q12 to 12qter)pat.

04q270   Negative band

Knorr-Gartner, H., Knorr, K. and Haas, B.: Inherited translocation t(4q-;18q+) with unbalanced progeny of different types. Humangenetik 21:315-321, 1974.
46,XX and XY,t(4;18)(q27;q21).
46,XX and XY,t(4;18)(4pter to 4q27::18q21 to 18qter;18pter to 18q21::4q27 to 4qter).
46,XX and XY,der(4)der(18)t(4;18)(q27;q21)mat and

pat.
46,XY,-18,+der(18)t(4;18)(q27;q21)mat.
46,XY,-18,+der(18)t(4;18)(18pter   to   18q21::4q27
to 4qter)mat.

04q280   Positive band

Jacobs, P. A., Buckton, K. E., Cunningham, C. and
Newton, M. S.: An analysis of the break points
of structural rearrangements in man. J. Med.
Genet. 11:50-64, 1974.
M. R. C. Registry No. K189-267-71 in this report.
46,XX,t(4;9)(q28;p2).

04q300

Same entry as in 04p100 (Bobrow, Jones and
Clarke, 1971).

Bobrow, M., Madan, K. and Pearson, P. L.:
Staining of some specific regions of human
chromosomes, particularly the secondary constriction of No. 9. Nature (New Biol.) 238:122-124,
1972.
46,XX or XY,t(4;9)(q3;q12).
46,XX or XY,t(4;9)(4pter to 4q3::9q12 to
9qter;9pter to 9q12::4q3 to 4qter).

Chesler, E., Freeman, I., Rosen, E. and Wilton,
E.: Congenital aneurysm of the membranous
ventricular septum associated with partial
trisomy E syndrome. Amer. Heart J. 79:805-810,
1970.
46,XX,t(4;18)(q3;q1).
Case N.L. in this report.
46,XX,-4,-der(4)t(4;18)(q3;q1)mat.
46,XX,-4,+der(4)t(4;18)(4pter to 4q3::18q1 to
18qter)mat.

Francke, U.: Quinacrine mustard fluorescence of
human chromosomes: characterization of unusual
translocations. Amer. J. Hum. Genet. 24:189-213,
1972.
46,XX,t(4;11)(q3;q).
Case No. 9: CJ 121468 in this report.
46,XX,-4,+der(4)t(4;11)(q3;q)mat.

Golbus, M. S., Conte, F. A. and Daentl, D. L.:

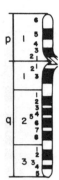

Deletion from the long arm of chromosome 4(46,XX,4q-) associated with congenital anomalies. J. Med. Genet. 10:82-84, 1973.
46,XX,del(4)(q3).
46,XX,del(4)(pter to q3:).

04q310   Negative band

Same entry as in 02q130 (German and Chaganti, 1973).

Jenkins, E. C., Curcuru-Giordano, F. M. and Krishna, S. G.: A case report of 46,XX,t(4;13)(q31;q14).   Newport Beach, Calif., Birth Defects Conf., National Foundation - March of Dimes, p. 135, June 16-21, 1974.
46,XX,t(4;13)(q31;q14).

Same entry as in 01p320 (Marsh et al., 1974).

04q340   Positive band

Same entry as in 04p120 (Lozzio and Klepper, 1974).

04q350   Negative band

Buckton, K. E.:   The identification of whole chromosomes or parts of chromosomes by the new banding techniques. Nobel Symposium 23:196-200, 1972.
46,XX,t(4;10)(q35;q23).
46,XX,-4,+der(4)t(4;10)(q35;q23)mat.

Same entry as in 04p130 (Dallapiccola et al., 1974).

de la Chapelle, A. and Schroder, J.: Autoradiographically identified karyotype 49,XXXXY,t(4;11)(q35;q23) confirmed by banding. Hereditas 74:291-292, 1973.
49,XXXXY,t(4;11)(q35;q23).
49,XXXXY,t(4;11)(4pter to 4q35::11q23 to 11qter;11pter to 11q23::?).
Mutant Cell Repository No. GM-157.

Dutrillaux, B., Jonasson, J., Lauren, K., Lejeune, J., Lindsten, J., Petersen, G. B. and

Saldana-Garcia, P.: An unbalanced 4q/21q translocation identified by the R but not by the G and
Q chromosome banding techniques. Ann. Genet.
16:11-16, 1973.
45,XY,-21,+t(4;21)(q35;q22).
45,XY,-21,+t(4;21)(4pter to 4q35::21q22 to
21qter).

Kreiger, D., Palmer, C. and Biegel, A.: Human
autosomal deletion mapping and HL-A. Humangenetik 23:159-160, 1974.
46,XY,t(4;?)(q35:?).

Same entry as in 02p210 (Lozzio and Klepper,
1974).

Ockey, C. H. and de la Chapelle, A.: Audioradio-
graphic reappraisal of an XXXxY male as a probable XXXXY with a 4-11 translocation. Cytogenetics 6:178-192, 1967.
46,XY,t(4;11)(q35;q23).
46,XY,der(4)der(11)t(4;11)(q35;q23)pat.
49,XXXXY,der(4)der(11)t(4;11)(q35;q23)pat.
49,XXXXY,der(4)der(11)t(4;11)(4pter to
4q35::11q23 to 11qter;11pter to 11q23::4q35 to
4qter)pat.
Mutant Cell Repository No. GM-157.

Same entry as in 04p140 (Rethore et al., 1974).

05p100

Same entry as in 02q000 (Bijlsma et al., 1971).

Bochkov, N. P., Kuleshov, N. P., Chebotarev, A.
N., Alekhin, V. I. and Midian, S. A.: Population
cytogenetic investigation of newborns in Moscow.
Humangenetik 22:139-152, 1974.
46,XY,inv(5)(pq).
46,XY,der(5)inv(5)(pq)pat.

Borgaonkar, D. S.: Application of new technics
of chromosome identification to cytogenetic
problems. Birth Defects: Original Article Series
9 No. 1:171-182, 1973.
46,XY,del(5)(p1).
46,XY,del(5)(qter to p1:).
It was shown that the terminal portion was

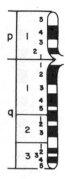

deleted from a chromosome No. 5 in a patient with the cri-du-chat syndrome.

Breg, W. R.: 1973.
46,XX,del(5)(p1).
46,XX,del(5)(qter to p1:).
Mutant Cell Repository No. GM-71.

Breg, W. R., Miller, D. A., Allderdice, P. W. and Miller, O. J.: Identification of translocation chromosomes by quinacrine fluorescence. Amer. J. Dis. Child. 123:561-564, 1972.
46,XX,t(5p-;14q+).
Patient 4 in this report.
Three mentally retarded offspring: one partially monosomic and two partially trisomic for the short arm of chromosome No. 5.

Breg, W. R., Steele, M. W., Miller, O. J., Warburton, D., de Capoa, A. and Allderdice, P. W.: The cri du chat syndrome in adolescents and adults: Clinical finding in 13 older patients with partial deletion of the short arm of chromo-some No. 5(5p-). J. Pediat. 77:782-791, 1970.
46,XX and XY,5p-.

Carpentier, S., Dutrillaux, B., Lafourcade, J., Berger, R., Rethore, M. O. and Lejeune, J.: Familial segregation of a t(5p-;13q+). A comple-mentary study from specimens stored in liquid nitrogen. Ann. Genet. 15:57-60, 1972.
46,XY,t(5p-;13q+).
46,XX,der(5)der(13)t(5p-;13q+)mat and pat.
46,XX and XY,-5,+der(5)t(5p-;13q+)mat.
46,XX,-13,+der(13)t(5p-;13q+)mat.

Carrel, R. E., Sparkes, R. S. and Wright, S. W.: Chromosome survey of moderately to profoundly retarded patients. Amer. J. Ment. Defic. 47:616-622, 1973.
46,XX,5p-/46,XX,r(5).

Caspersson, T., Lindsten, J. and Zech, L.: Identification of the abnormal B group chromosome in the "cri-du-chat" syndrome by Q-M fluores-cence. Exp. Cell Res. 61:475-476, 1970.
46,XX,del(5)(p1).
46,XX,del(5)(qter to p1:).

A portion of the short arm of chromosome No. 5 is deleted in patients with what has been called the 'cat's cry syndrome' because of the similarity with the mewing-like cry during infancy.

p | 1 | 5 4 3 2

q | 1 2 3 4 5 | 2 1 2 3 | 3 3 1 2 4 5 6

Catti, A. and Schmid, W.: A pericentric inversion, 5p-q+, and additional complex rearrangements in a case of cri-du-chat syndrome. Cytogenetics 10:50-60, 1971.
46,XX,inv(5)(pq),15q+,r(C).
Chromosome identification by autoradiography.

Cohen, M. M., Lin, C. C. and Davidson, R. G.: Two B-C translocations specifically identified by 'banding' techniques. J. Med. 3:216-223, 1972.
Patient B. G. in this report.
46,XY,t(5p+;6q-).

DeGeorge, F. V., Neu, R. L. and Gardner, L. I.: A t(5p-;21q+) in a family with Down's syndrome. Amer. J. Hum. Genet. 26:25A, 1974.
46,XX,t(5p-;21q+).

Dutrillaux, B.: Chromosomal aspects of human male sterility. Nobel Symposium 23:205-208, 1972.
46,XY,t(5;8)(p1;q1).
46,XY,t(5;8)(5qter to 5p1::8q1 to 8qter;8pter to 8q1::5p1 to 5pter).

Ferguson-Smith, M. A.: Human chromosomes in meiosis. In Human Genetics, pp. 195-211. Ed. by de Grouchy, J., Ebbing, F. J. C. and Henderson, I. W., Amsterdam Excerpta Medica, 1972.
46,XY,t(5;10)(p1;q).

Same entry as in 04q000 (Grotsky, Hsu and Hirschhorn, 1971).

Guttler, F. and Niebuhr, E.: On the possible localization of a gene for triosephosphate isomerase on the short arm of human chromosome 5. Humangenetik 17:301-306, 1973.

James, A. E., Atkins, L., Feingold, M. and Janower, M. L.: The cri du chat syndrome. Radiology 92:50-52, 1969.
46,XX and XY,5p-.

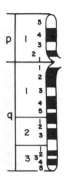

Kadotani, T., Ohama, K., Sofuni, T. and Hamilton, H. B.: Aberrant karyotypes and spontaneous abortion in a Japanese family. Nature 225:735, 1970.
46,XX and XY,t(?5;?11)(p1;q2).
Chromosome identification by autoradiography.

Same entry as in 01q000 (Leisti, 1971).

Lejeune, J., Lafourcade, J., Berger, R., Vialatte, J., Boeswillwald, M., Seringe, P. and Turpin, R.: Trois cas de deletion partielle du bras court d'un chromosome 5. C. R. Acad. Sci. 257:3098-3102, 1963.
46,XX and XY,del(5)(p1).
46,XX and XY,del(5)(qter to p1:).
The cri-du-chat syndrome was first described in this report.

Lubs, H. A. and Lubs, M. L.: Studies of newborns in Grand Junction, Colorado. Twelfth Ann. Somatic Cell Genet. Conf., Utah, 78-79, 1974.
46,XY,t(5p+;10q-).

Mann, J. and Rafferty, J. H.: Cri-du-chat syndrome combined with partial C-group trisomy. J. Med. Genet. 9:289-292, 1972.
46,XX,t(5;11)(p1;q1).
46,XX,t(5;11)(5qter to 5p1::11q1 to 11qter;11pter to 11q1::5p1 to 5pter).
46,XY,der(5)der(11)t(5;11)(p1;q1)mat.
46,XX,-5,+der(5)t(5;11)(p1;q1)pat.
46,XX,-5,+der(5)t(5;11)(5qter to 5p1::11q1 to 11qter)pat.

Miller, D. A., Allderdice, P. W., Miller, O. J. and Breg, W. R.: Quinacrine fluorescence patterns of human D group chromosomes. Nature 232:24-27, 1971.
46,XY,t(5;14)(p;q).

Newton, M. S., Cunningham, C., Jacobs, P. A., Price, W. H. and Fraser, I. A.: Chromosome survey of a hospital for the mentally subnormal. Part 2: Autosome abnormalities. Clin. Genet. 3:226-248, 1972.
M. R. C. Registry No. K156-278-67 in this report.
46,XX,del(5)(p1).

46,XX,del(5)(qter to p1:).

Niebuhr, E.: A 45,XX,5-,13-,dic+ karyotype in a
case of cri-du-chat syndrome. Cytogenetics
11:165-177, 1972.
45,XX,tdic(5;13)(p1;p1),mar16.
45,XX,tdic(5;13)(5qter to 5p1::13p1 to
13qter),mar16.

Opitz, J. M. and Patau, K.: The partial trisomy
5p syndrome. Newport Beach, Calif., Birth
Defects Conf., National Foundation - March of
Dimes, p. 85, June 16-21, 1974.
46,XX,t(5;12)(p1;q).
46,XX,t(5;12)(5qter to 5p1::12q to 12qter;12pter
to 12q::5p1 to 5pter).
46,XX,der(5)der(12)t(5;12)(p1;q)mat.
46,XX,-12,+der(12)t(5;12)(p1;q)mat.
46,XX,-12,+der(12)t(5;12)(12pter to 12q::5p1 to
5pter)mat.

Singer, H. and Scaife, N.: Simultaneous occurrence of ring "G" chromosome and group "B"
pericentric inversion in the same individual:
Case report and review of the literature.
Pediatrics 46:74-83, 1970.
46,XY,inv(5)(pq),r(21).

Singh, D. N., Osborne, R. A. and Wiscovitch, R.
A.: Transmission of the cri-du-chat syndrome
from a maternal balanced translocation carrier,
t(5p-;11q+). Humangenetik 20:361-365, 1973.
46,XX,t(5;11)(p1;q2).
46,XX,t(5;11)(5qter to 5p1::11q2 to 11qter;11pter
to 11q2::5p1 to 5pter).
46,XY,-5,+der(5)t(5;11)(p1;q2)mat.
46,XY,-5,+der(5)t(5;11)(5qter to 5p1::11q2 to
11qter)mat.

Same entry as in 04p100 (Taillemite et al.,
1973).

Vuorenkoski, V., Lind, J., Partanen, T. J.,
Lejeune, J., Lafourcade, J. and Wasz-Hockert, O.:
Spectrographic analysis of cries from children
with maladie du cri du chat. Ann. Paediat. Fenn.
12:174-180, 1966.

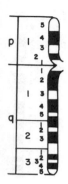

White, B. J., Van de Water, L. and Tjio, J. H.: A family with balanced translocation, t(5p-;6p+). J. Med. Genet. 8:188-194, 1971.
46,XX,t(5p-;6p+).
Chromosome identification by autoradiography.

Wolf, U., Reinwein, H., Gey, W. and Klose, J.: Cri-du-chat-syndrom mit translokation 5/D2. Humangenetik 2:63-77, 1966.
45,XX,-5,-14,+t(5;?14)(p1;q).
45,XX,-5,-14,+t(5;?14)(5qter to 5p1::14q to 14qter).

05p110   Negative band

Jacobs, P. A., Buckton, K. E., Cunningham, C. and Newton, M. S.: An analysis of the break points of structural rearrangements in man. J. Med. Genet. 11:50-64, 1974.
M. R. C. Registry No. K149-177-69 in this report.
46,XY,t(5;11)(p11;p15).

05p130   Negative band

Faed, M. J. W., Marrian, V. J., Robertson, J., Robson, E. B. and Cook, P. J. L.: Inherited pericentric inversion of chromosome 5: A family with history of neonatal death and a case of the "cri du chat" syndrome. Cytogenetics 11:400-411, 1972.
46,XX and XY,inv(5)(p13q33).
46,XX and XY,inv(5)(5pter to 5p13::q33 to p13::q33 to qter)
46,XY,der(5)inv(5)(p13q33)mat.

Friedrich, U. and Nielsen, J.: Autosomal deletions 46,XY,del(12)(p11) and 46,XY/
46,XY,del(5)(p13) with no effect on physical or mental development. Humangenetik 21:127-132, 1974.
Proband No. 7255 in this report.
46,XY/46,XY,del(5)(p13).
46,XY/46,XY,del(5)(qter to p13:).

Jacobs, P. A., Buckton, K. E., Cunningham, C. and Newton, M. S.: An analysis of the break points of structural rearrangements in man. J. Med. Genet. 11:50-64, 1974.

M. R. C. Registry No. K96-82-69 in this report.
46,XY,inv(5)(p13q13).
46,XY,inv(5)(pter to p13::q13 to p13::q13 to qter).

05p140   Positive band

Berger, R., Tonati, G., Derre, J., Ortiz, M. A. and Martinetti, J.: "Cri du chat" syndrome with maternal insertional translocation. Clin. Genet. 5:428-432, 1974.
46,XX,ins(17;5)(q21;p14p15).
46,XX,ins(17;5)(17pter to 17q12::5p14 to 5p15::17q21 to 17qter).

Borgaonkar, D. S., Blair, S. M., Lutz, J. B., Kelly, T. E., Tice, R. R., Delaney, N. V., Hutchinson, J. R. and Bias, W. B.: Cytogenetic study of a 5/14 translocation in man. J. Hered. 64:299-300. 1973.
46,XY,t(5;14)(p14;q21).
46,XY,t(5;14)(5pter to 5p14::14q21 to 14qter;14pter to 14q21::5p14 to 5pter).
46,XX and XY,der(5)der(14)t(5;14)(p14;q21)mat and pat.
Transmission of the reciprocal translocation through three generations is documented in this report.
Mutant Cell Repository No. GM-589.

Kreiger, D., Palmer, C. and Biegel, A.: Human autosomal deletion mapping and HL-A. Humangenetik 23:159-160, 1974.
46,XX,del(5)(p14).
46,XX,del(5)(qter to p14:).

Same entry as in 01q430 (Martinetti and Noel, 1973).

Niebuhr, E.: Localization of the deleted segment in the cri-du-chat syndrome. Humangenetik 16:357-358, 1972.
46,XY,t(5;22)(p14;p1).
46,XX and XY,-5,+der(5)t(5;22)(p14;p1)pat.
The author suggests that 05p140 and 05p150 are the pathogenetic segments for the cri du chat syndrome.

05p150   Negative band

Same entry as in 05p140 (Berger et al., 1974).

Dewald, G. W., Spurbeck, J. and Gordon, H.:
Automated videodensitometric analysis of autosomal translocations. Amer. J. Hum. Genet.
26:26A, 1974.
Family B in this report.
46,XX and XY,t(5;12)(p15;p11).

Nakagome, Y., Iinuma, K. and Taniguchi, K.:
Points of exchange in a human No. 5 ring chromosome. Cytogenet. Cell Genet. 12:35-39, 1973.
46,XYq+,r(5)(p15q35).
46,XYq+,r(5)(p15 to q35).
The Y chromosome was as long as a D group chromosome.   It was estimated that about 5.5% of the
chromosome 5 material has been lost due to the
ring formation in a patient with cri-du-chat
syndrome.

Same entry as in 05p140 (Niebuhr, 1972).

05q000

Same entry as in 05p100 (Bochkov et al., 1974).

Same entry as in 05p130 (Faed et al., 1972).

Same entry as in 01q000 (Ferguson-Smith, 1974).

Fredga, K. and Hall, B.:   A complex familial
translocation involving chromosomes 5, 9 and 13.
Cytogenetics 9:294-306, 1970.
46,XX,t(5;9;13)(q;p;q).
46,XX,t(5;9;13)(5pter to 5q::13q to 13qter;9qter
to 9p::5q to 5qter;13pter to 13q::9p to 9pter.
46,XX,der(5)der(9)der(13)t(5;9;13)(q;p;q)mat.

Lindenbaum, R. H. and Butler, L. J.: Child with
multiple anomalies and a group B(4-5) long arm
deletion (Bq-).   Arch. Dis. Child. 46:99-101,
1971.
46,XY,del(5)(q).
46,XY,del(5)(pter to q:).

Lubs, H. A. and Lubs, M. L.: Studies of newborns

in Grand Junction, Colorado. Twelfth Ann. Somatic Cell Genet. Conf. Utah, 78-79, 1974. 46,t(5q-;11q+).

Same entry as in 0Xq000 (Mann and Higgins, 1974).

Same entry as in 030000 (Neu and Gardner, 1972).

Rudd, N. L. and Lamarche, P. H.: Gene deletion and duplication effects on phenotype and gamma globulin levels. J. Med. Genet. 8:97-106, 1971. 46,XX,t(?5q+;?18q-). 46,XX and XY,-5,+der(5)t(?5q+;?18q-)mat. 46,XY,-18,+der(18)t(?5q+;?18q-)mat.

05q100

Knight, L. A., Sakaguchi, S. and Luzzatti, L.: Unusual mechanism of transmission of a maternal chromosome translocation. Amer. J. Dis. Child. 121:162-167, 1971. 46,XX,t(5;14)(q1;p1). 46,XX,t(5;14)(5pter to 5q1::14p1 to 14pter;14qter to 14p1::5q1 to 5qter). 46,XX,-5,+der(5)t(5;14)(q1;p1)mat. 46,XX,-5,+der(5)t(5;14)(5pter to 5q1::14p1 to 14pter)mat.

05q110   Negative band

Leisti, J.: "Cri du chat" and "Trisomy 13" syndromes in an infant with an urbalanced chromosomal translocation. Newport Beach, Calif., Birth Defects Conf., National Foundation - March of Dimes, p. 195, June 16-21, 1974. 46,XX,t(5;13)(q11;p11). Case HH 613318 in this report. 46,XX,-5,+der(13)t(5;13)(q11;p11)mat. 46,XX,-5,+der(13)t(5;13)(13qter to 13p11::5q11 to 5qter)mat.

05q120   Positive band

van den Berghe, H., Cassiman, J. J., David, G., Fryns, J. P., Michaux, J. L. and Sokal, G.: Distinct haematological disorder with deletion of the long arm of No. 5 chromosome. Nature 251:437-438, 1974.

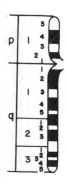

46,XX and XY,del(5)(q12 to 15 and q21 to 23).
46,XX and XY,del(5)(pter to q12::5q21 to qter).
The hematological disorder is characterized by longstanding aregenerative slightly macrocytic anemia.   Two females and one male were studied. The chromosome abnormality was found in bone marrow cells cultured without phytohemagglutinin.

05q130   Negative band

Same entry as in 05p130 (Jacobs et al., 1974).

05q150   Negative band

Same entry as in 01q430 (Martinetti and Noel, 1973).

Same entry as in 05q120 (van den Berghe et al., 1974).

05q200

Jacobs, P. A., Buckton, K. E., Cunningham, C. and Newton, M. S.: An analysis of the break points of structural rearrangements in man. J. Med. Genet. 11:50-64, 1974.
M. R. C. Registry No. K73-283-69 in this report.
46,XY,t(5;16)(q2;p13).

05q210   Positive band

Same entry as in 05q120 (van den Berghe et al., 1974).

05q230   Positive band

Same entry as in 05q120 (van den Berghe et al., 1974).

05q300

Same entry as in 02p100 (Lundsten, Vestermark and Philip, 1974).

05q310   Negative band

Same entry as in 02p230 (Ferguson-Smith et al., 1973).

05q330   Negative band

Same entry as in 05p130 (Faed et al., 1972).

Hirschhorn, K., Lucas, M. and Wallace, I.:
Precise identification of various chromosomal
abnormalities.   Ann. Hum. Genet.   36:375-379,
1973.
Family La(Gc 765) in this report.
46,XX,t(5;10)(q33;q11).
See Lucas and Wallace (1972) in entry 05q330.

Lucas, M. and Wallace, I.: Recurrent abortions
and chromosome abnormalities. J. Obstet. Gynaec.
Brit. Comm. 79:1119-1127, 1972.
Family La in this report.
46,XX,t(5;10)(q33;q11).
46,XX,t(5;10)(5pter to 5q33::10q11 to 10qter;10p-
ter to 10q11::5q33 to 5qter).
47,XX,+14,der(5)der(10)t(5;10)(q33;q11)mat.
See Hirschhorn, Lucas and Wallace (1973) in entry
05q330.

05q350   Negative band

Boue, J. and Boue, A.: L'interet en diagnostic
prenatal des techniques nouvelles d'identification chromosomique dans des translocations et une
aneusomie de recombinaison. Nouv. Presse Med.
2:3097-3102, 1973.
Observation No. 1094 in this report.
46,XX,t(5;10)(q35;q22).

Kreiger, D., Palmer, C. and Biegel, A.: Human
autosomal deletion mapping and HL-A. Humangenetik 23:159-160, 1974.
46,XY,t(5;?)(q35;?).

Same entry as in 05p150 (Nakagome, Iinuma and
Taniguchi, 1973).

060000

Same entry as in 020000 (Breg et al., 1972).

Jacobs, P. A., Buckton, K. E., Cunningham, C. and
Newton, M. S.: An analysis of the break points
of structural rearrangements in man. J. Med.

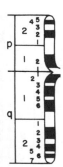

Genet. 11:50-64, 1974.
46,XX,t(6p14p)t(6q14q).
M. R. C. Registry No. K138-3-71 in this report.
46,XX,der(6)der(14)t(6p14p)t(6q14q)mat.

06p000

Jacobsen, P., Mikkelsen, M., Niebuhr, E. and de
Grouchy, J.: A case of 18q- in a t(18q-;6p+)
family. Ann. Genet. 14:41-48, 1971.
46,XX and XY,t(6p+;18q-).
46,XY,der(6)der(18)t(6p+;18q-)mat.
46,XY,-18,+der(18)t(6p+;18q-)pat.

Moore, C. M., Heller, R. H. and Thomas, G. H.:
Developmental abnormalities associated with a
ring chromosome 6. J. Med. Genet. 10:299-303,
1973.
46,XX,r(6)(pq).
Mutant Cell Repository No. GM-109.

van den Berghe, H., Fryns, J. P., Cassiman, J. J.
and David, G.: Ring chromosome 6. Karyotype
46,XY,r(6)/45,XY,-6. Ann. Genet. 17:29-35, 1974.
46,XY,r(6)/45,XY,-6.

Wright, Y. M., Clark, W. E. and Breg, W. R.:
Craniorachischisis in a partially trisomic 11
fetus in a family with reproductive failure and a
reciprocal translocation, t(6p+;11q-). J. Med.
Genet. 11:69-75, 1974.
46,XY,t(6p+;11q-).
46,XY,-6,der(6p+)pat.

06p110   Negative band

de Grouchy, J., Veslot, J., Bonnette, J. and
Roidot, M.: A case of ?6p- chromosomal aberration. Amer. J. Dis. Child. 115:93-99, 1973.
46,XY,6p-.

Jacobs, P. A., Buckton, K. E., Cunningham, C. and
Newton, M. S.: An analysis of the break points
of structural rearrangements in man. J. Med.
Genet. 11:50-64, 1974.
M. R. C. Registry No. K55-137-68 in this report.
46,XX,t(6;13)(p11;q12).

Same entry as in 04p160 (Jacobs et al., 1974).

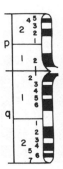

06p200

Lam, L. U.: Rotterdam Conference, 1974.
46,XX and XY,inv(6)(p22 or 23q22 or 23).
46,XX and XY,der(6)inv(6)mat.

06p220   Positive band

Gouw, W. L., ten Kate, L. P. and Anders, G. J. P.
A.:   A case of 18q-   in a family with a translocation   t(6p+;18q-),   identified by the Giemsa-
banding technique.   Humangenetik   19:123-126,
1973.
46,XX,t(6;18)(p22;q12).
46,XX,t(6;18)(6qter to 6p22::18q12 to 18qter;18p-
ter to 18q12::6p22 to 6pter).
46,XX,der(6)der(18)t(6;18)(p22;q12)mat.
46,XY,-18,+der(18)t(6;18)(p22;q12)mat.
46,XY,-18,+der(18)t(6;18)(18pter   to   18q12::6p22
to 6pter)mat.

06p230   Negative band

Same entry as in 02q130 (Kreiger, Palmer and
Biegel, 1974).

06p250   Negative band

Borgaonkar, D. S., Bias, W. B., Chase, G. A.,
Sadasivan, G., Herr, H. M., Golomb, H. M., Bahr,
G. F. and Kunkel, L. M.: Identification of a C6/
G21 translocation chromosome by the Q-M and
Giemsa banding techniques in a patient with
Down's syndrome, with possible assignment of Gm
locus. Clin. Genet. 4:53-57, 1973.
45,XX,-6,-21+t(6;21)(p25;q11).
45,XX,-6,-21,+t(6;21)(6qter   to   6p25::21q11   to
21qter).
46,XX,-6,+der(6)t(6;21)(p25;q11)mat.
Mutant Cell Repository No. GM-144.
45,XY,-6,-21,+der(6)t(6;21)(p25;q11)mat.

Borgaonkar, D. S., Greene, A. E., and Coriell, L.
L.:   A (6;21) translocation, unbalanced, 46
chromosomes: Repository identification No. GM-
144. Cytogenet. Cell Genet. 13:403-405, 1974.

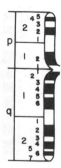

Lejeune, J.: Scientific impact of the study of fine structure of chromatids. Nobel Symposium 23:16-24, 1973.

Pallister, P. D., Patau, K., Inhorn, S. L. and Opitz, J. M.: A woman with multiple congenital anomalies, mental retardation and mosaicism for an unusual translocation chromosome t(6;19). Clin. Genet. 5:188-195, 1974.
Patient MH 211129 in this report.
45,XX,-6,-19,+t(6;19)(p25;p13).
45,XX,-6,-19,+t(6;19)(6qter to 6p25::19p13 to 19qter).
The centromere of chromosome No. 6 is inactivated.

Rethore, M. O., Larget-Piet, L., Abonyi, D., Boeswillwald, M., Berger, R., Carpentier, S., Cruveiller, J., Dutrillaux, B., Lafourcade, J., Penneau, M. and Lejeune, J.: Sur quatre cas de trisomie pour le bras court du chromosome 9. Individualisation d'une nouvelle entite morbide. Ann. Genet. 13:217-232, 1970.
46,XX,rcp(6;9)(p25;q12).
46,XX,rcp(6;9)(6qter to 6p25::9q12 to 9qter;9pter to 9q12::6p25 to 6pter).
47,XX,+der(9)t(6;9)(p25;q12)mat.
47,XX,+der(9)t(6;9)(9pter to 9q12::6p25 to 6pter)mat.
Additional information was obtained from the article by Lejeune (1973) cited in 06p250.

06q000

Same entry as in 05p100 (Cohen, Lin and Davidson, 1972).

Same entry as in 01q230 (Dewald, Spurbeck and Gordon, 1974).

Same entry as in 0Yq100 (Leisti, 1971).

06q100

Jacobs, P. A., Buckton, K. E., Cunningham, C. and Newton, M. S.: An analysis of the break points of structural rearrangements in man. J. Med. Genet. 11:50-64, 1974.

M. R. C. Registry No. K47-78-68 in this report.
46,XY,t(6;12)(q1;q24).

Rohde, R. A. and Catz, B.:   Maternal transmission
of a new group -C(6/9) chromosomal syndrome.
Lancet 1:838-840, 1964.
46,XX,t(6;9)(q1;q3).

06q200

Francke, U.:   Quinacrine mustard fluorescence of
human chromosomes: characterization of unusual
translocations.   Amer. J. Hum. Genet. 24:189-213,
1972.
Case 3: LB 220660 in this report.
46,XY,t(6;12)(q2;q).

Fryns, J. P., Eggermont, E., Verresen, H. and van
den Berghe, H.:   Partial trisomy 13: Karyotype
46,XY,-6,+t(13q6q). Humangenetik 21:47-54, 1974.
46,XY,-6,+t(6;13)(q2;q).
46,XY,-6,+t(6;13)(6pter to 6q2::13q to 13qter).

Fryns, J. P., van Herck, G., Cassiman, J. J. and
van den Berghe, H.:   Trisomy 12p due to familial
t(12p-,6q+)   translocation.   Humangenetik 24:247-
252, 1974.
46,XY,t(6;12)(q2;p11).
47,XY,-6,+der(6)t(6;12)(q2;p11)pat.

Nakagome, Y., Iinuma, K. and Matsui, I.:   Three
translocations involving C- or G-group chromosomes. J. Med. Genet. 10:174-176, 1973.
Case A in this report.
46,XX,t(6;18)(q2;q1).
46,XX,t(6;18)(6pter to 6q2::18q1 to 18qter;18pter
to 18q1::6q2 to 6qter).
46,XX and XY,der(16)der(18)t(6;18)(q2;q1)mat.
46,XX and XY,-6,+der(6)t(6;18)(q2;q1)mat.
46,XX and XY,-6,+der(6)t(6;18)(6pter to 6q2::18q1
to 18qter)mat.

06q210   Negative band

Allderdice, P. W., Miller, O. J., Miller, D. A.,
Breg, W. R., Gendal, E. and Zelson, C.: Familial
translocation involving chromosomes 6,14, and 20
identified by quinacrine fluorescence. Human-

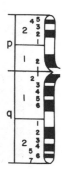

genetik 13:205-209, 1971.
46,XX,t(6;14;20)(q21;q2;p1).
46,XX,t(6;14;20)(6pter to 6q21;14pter to 14q2::6q21 to 6qter;20qter to 20p1::14q2 to 14qter).
47,XX,-6,+der(6)+der(14)t(6;14;20)(q21;q2;p1).
47,XX,-6,+der(6)+der(14)t(6;14;20)(6pter to 6q21;14pter to 14q2::6q21 to 6qter).

Klinger, H. P.: Personal Communication, 1974.
46,XX,t(6;18)(q21;p11).
Mutant Cell Repository No. GM-610.

Thurmon, T. F., Robertson, K. P. and Campbell, M. C.: Acrocephalosyndactyly and partial trisomies. Newport Beach, Calif., Birth Defects Conf., National Foundation - March of Dimes, p. 96, June 16-21, 1974.
46,XX,t(6;10)(q21;q).
46,XX,t(6;10)(6pter to 6q21g;10pter to 10qter::6q21 to 6qter).
46,XX,-10,+der(10)t(6;10)(10pter .to 10qter::6q21 to 6qter)mat.
The authors imply that only one break occurred to form the translocation chromosome.

06q250   Negative band

Mikkelsen, M. and Dyggve, H.: (6;15) Transloca-tion with loss of chromosome material in the patient and various chromosome aberrations in family members. Humangenetik 18:195-202, 1973.
45,XY,tan(6;15)(q25;q12).
45,XY,tan(6;15)(6pter to 6q25::15q12 to 15pter).

06q270   Negative band

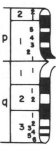

Niebuhr, E.: A familial translocation t(6q+;8q-) identified by fluorescence microscopy. Human-genetik 18:189-192, 1973.
46,XX,t(6;8)(q27;q12).
46,XX and XY,der(6)der(8)t(6;8)(q27;q12)mat.

070000

Same entry as in 020000 (Jacobs et al., 1974).

07p000

Breg, W. R., Allderdice, P. W., Miller, D. A. and
Miller, O. J.: Quinacrine fluorescence patterns
and terminal DNA labelling of human C group
chromosomes. Nature (New Biol.) 236:76-78, 1972.
Case No. JC 091069 in this report.
46,XY,r(7).

Caspersson, T., Hulten, M., Lindsten, J. and
Zech, L.:   Chromatid interchange resulting in
duplication of the short arm of chromosome number
7 in man. Ann. Genet. 14:142-144, 1971.
46,XX/46,XX,dup(7)(p).

Same entry as in 04q000 (Cohen, Lin and Davidson,
1972).

Dutrillaux, B.:   Chromosomal aspects of human
male sterility.   Nobel Symposium 23:205-208,
1972.
46,XY,inv(7)(pq).

Wilson, M. G., Fujimoto, A., Shinno, N. W. and
Towner, J. W.:   Giant satellites or translocation? Cytogenet. Cell Genet. 12:209-214, 1973.
46,XX,t(7p-;13s+).

07p100

Noel, B., Mottet, J., Nantois, Y. and Quack, B.:
Contribution a l'identification du petit chromosome submetacentrique surnumeraire dans le
syndrome des yeux de chat. J. Genet. Hum. 21:23-
32, 1973.
del(7)(p1q11).
del(7)(:p1 to cen to q1:).

07p130   Negative band

Cooledge, J. W., Beatty-DeSana, J. W. and Hoggard, M. J.: The occurrence of a translocation
(7;14) which has been associated with ataxia-
telangiectasia in cytogenetic studies of spontaneous chromosomal aberrations in human leuco-
cyte culture. Amer. J. Hum. Genet. 26:23A, 1974.
46,XX,t(7;14)(p13;q12q13).

Same entry as in 02p250 (Subrt, Kozak and Hnikova, 1973).

07p140   Positive band

Same entry as in 02p250 (Subrt, Kozak and Hnikova, 1973).

07p200

Miller, R., Coriell, L. L. and Greene, A. E.:
Personal communication, 1974.
46,XY,t(7;10)(p2;q11).
46,XY,t(7;10)(7qter to 7p2:10q11 to 10qter;10pter
to 10q11::7p2 to 7pter).
Mutant Cell Repository No. GM-44.

07p220   Negative band

Schleiermacher, E., Schliebitz, U., Steffens, C.,
Ronipe, G. and Schmidt, U.: Brother and sister
with trisomy 10p: a new syndrome. Humangenetik
23:163-172, 1974.
46,XX,t(7;10)(p22;p11).
46,XX,t(7;10)(7qter to 7p22::10p11 to 10pter;10q-
ter to 10p11::7p22 to 7pter).
46,XX,der(7)der(10)t(7;10)(p22;p11)mat.
46,XX and XY,-7,+der(7)t(7;10)(p22;p11)mat.
46,XX and XY,-7,+der(7)t(7;10)(7qter to
7p22::10p11 to 10pter)mat.
Both of these children are trisomic for the short
arm of chromosome 10.

Zachai, E. H. and Breg, W. R.: Ring chromosome 7
with variable phenotypic expression. Cytogenet.
Cell Genet. 12:40-48, 1973.
Cases 1 and 2 in this report.
45,XY,/46,XY,r(7)(p22q36).
45,XY,-7/46,XY,r(7)(p22 to q36).

07q000

Same entry as in 07p000 (Dutrillaux, 1972).

Giraud, F., Hartung, M., Mattei, J. F. and
Mattei, M. G.: t(7q-;21q+) and familial trisomy
21. Ann. Genet. 17:49-53, 1974.
46,XX,t(7;21)(q;q2).
46,XX,t(7;21)(7pter to 7q::21q2 to 21qter;21pter
to 21q2::7q to 7qter).
47,XX and XY,-7,+der(7)+der(21)t(7;21)(q;q2)mat,+

21.

Same entry as in 02p000 (Handmaker, Hall and Conte, 1974).

Leisti, J.: Structural variation in human mitotic chromosomes. Ann. Acad. Sci. fenn. (Med.) Series A, IV, Biologica 179:1-69, 1971. Case No. 19 in this report.
46,XX,t(Cq-;Dq+),11qh.

Same entry as in 03p000 (Lejeune, 1973).

Newton, M. S., Cunningham, C., Jacobs, P. A., Price, W. H. and Fraser, I. A.: Chromosome survey of a hospital for the mentally subnormal. Part 2: Autosome abnormalities. Clin. Genet. 3:226-248, 1972.
46,XX,t(7q-;19q+).
M. R. C. Registry No. K43-279-67 in this report.
46,XX,-19,+der(19)t(7q-;19q+)mat.

Same entry as in 02p000 (Shokeir, Ying and Pabello, 1973).

07q110   Negative band

Jacobs, P. A., Buckton, K. E., Cunningham, C. and Newton, M. S.: An analysis of the break points of structural rearrangements in man. J. Med. Genet. 11:50-64, 1974.
M. R. C. Repository No. K78-153-70 in this report.
46,XX,t(7;11)(q11;q25).

Lozzio, C. B. and Klepper, M. B.: Chromosome aberrations identified by the new banding techniques. Amer. J. Hum. Genet. 26:55A, 1974.
t(7;14)(q11q32).
This new balanced translocation was found in a child.

Same entry as in 01p320 (Marsh et al., 1974).

Same entry as in 07p100 (Noel et al., 1973).

07q200

Same entry as in 03q200 (Altman, Palmer and Baehner, 1974).

07q220   Negative band

Carpentier, S., Rethore, M. O. and Lejeune, J.: Partial trisomy 7q due to familial translocation t(7;12)(q22;q24). Ann. Genet. 15:283-286, 1972.
46,XX,t(7;12)(q22;q24).
46,XX,t(7;12)(7pter to 7q22::12q24 to 12qter;12pter to 12q24::7q22 to 7qter).
46,XX,der(7)der(12)t(7;12)(q22;q24)mat.
Proposita in this report.
46,XY,-12,+der(12)t(7;12)(q22;q24).
46,XY,-12,+der(12)t(7;12)(12pter to 12q24::7q22 to 7qter).

Same entry as in 03q270 (Grace, Sutherland and Bain, 1972).

07q300

Bass, H. N., Crandall, B. F. and Marcy, S. M.: Two different chromosome abnormalities resulting from a translocation carrier father. J. Pediat. 83:1034-1038, 1973.
46,XY,t(7;21)(q3;q2).
46,XX,-7,+der(7)t(7;21)(q3;q2)pat.
Patient C.H. 081171 in this report.
46,XX,-21,+der(21)t(7;21)(q3;q2)pat.
46,XX,-21,+der(21)t(7;21)(21pter to 21q2::7q3 to 7qter)pat.

de la Chapelle, A., Schroder, J. and Kokkonen, J.: Cytogenetics of recurrent abortion or unsuccessful pregnancy. Int. J. Fertil. 18:215-219, 1973.
46,XX,t(7;14)(q3;q2).
46,XX and XY,-7,-14,+der(7)+
der(14)t(7;14)(q3;q2)mat.

Same entry as in 0Yq110 (Develing, Conte and Epstein, 1973).

07q310   Positive band

Alfi, O. S., Donnell, G. N. and Kramer, S. L.: Partial trisomy of the long arm of chromosome No.

7.   J. Med. Genet. 10:187-189, 1973.
46,XY,t(7;14)(q31;q32).
46,XY,-14,+der(14)t(7;14)(q31;q32)pat.
46,XY,-14,+der(14)t(7;14)(14pter   to   14q32::7q31
to 7qter)pat.

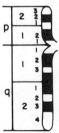

Same entry as in 03p210 (Rethore et al., 1972).

Vogel,   W.,   Siebers,   J.   W.   and   Reinwein,   H.:
Partial   trisomy   7q.   Ann.   Genet.   16:277-280,
1973.
46,XX,t(7;21)(q31;p13).
46,XX,-21,+der(21)t(7;21)(q31;p13)mat.
46,XX,-21,+der(21)t(7;21)(21qter   to   21p13::7q31
to 7qter)mat.

07q320   Negative band

Buckton,   K.   E.:   The   identification of whole
chromosomes   or   parts   of chromosomes by the new
banding   techniques.   Nobel Symposium 23:196-200,
1972.
46,XX,t(7;19)(q32;q13).
46,XX,-19,+der(19)t(7;19)(q32;q13)mat.

Same   entry   as   in 03q270 (Grace, Sutherland and
Bain, 1972).

Same entry as in 01p320 (Marsh et al., 1974).

Thompson, B. H. and Palmer, C. G.:   Familial 7,18
translocation.   Amer.   J.   Hum.   Genet. 26:87A,
1974.
46,XX,t(7;18)(q32;q23).
46,XX and XY,der(7)der(18)t(7;18)(q32;q23)mat and
pat.
Translocation found in three generations.

07q360   Negative band

Same entry as in 07p220 (Zachai and Breg, 1973).

08p000

Breg,   W.   R.,   Allderdice,   P.   W.,   Miller,   D.   A.   and
Miller,   O.   J.:   Quinacrine fluorescence patterns
and   terminal   DNA   labelling   of   human   C   group
chromosomes.   Nature (New Biol.) 236:76-78, 1972.

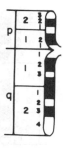

46,XY,inv(8)(pq).

Buckton, K. E.: The identification of whole chromosomes or parts of chromosomes by the new banding techniques. Nobel Symposium 23:196-200, 1972.
46,XX,t(8;18)(p;p11).

del Solar, C. and Uchida, I. A.: Identification of chromosomal abnormalities by quinacrine-staining technique in patients with normal karyotypes by conventional analysis. J. Pediat. 84:534-538, 1974.
See Uchida and Lin (1973) in entry 08p230.

German, J.: Studying chromosomes today. Amer. Sci. 58:182-201, 1970.
46,XX,inv(8)(pq).
46,XX and XY,der(8)inv(pq)mat.

Same entry as in 08+ (Lejeune and Rethore, 1973).

Pfeiffer, R. A. and Lenard, H. G.: Ring chromosom 8 (46,XY,8r) bei einem Jungen. Klin. Paediat. 185:187-191, 1973.
46,XY,r(8).

08p100

Rosenthal, I. M., Krompotic, E., Bocian, M. and Szego, K.: Trisomy of the short arm of chromosome 8: Association with translocation between chromosomes 8 and 22 46,XY,22-,t(8p22q)+. Clin. Genet. 4:507-516, 1973.
46,XX,t(8;22)(p1;p1).
46,XY,der(8)der(22)t(8;22)(p1;p1)mat.
46,XY,-22,+der(22)t(8;22)(p1;p1)mat.

08p110   Negative band

Jacobs, P. A., Buckton, K. E., Cunningham, C. and Newton, M. S.: An analysis of the break points of structural rearrangements in man. J. Med. Genet. 11:50-64, 1974.
M. R. C. Registry No. K199-202-70 in this report.
46,XX,t(8;15)(p11;q24 or 25 or 26).

08p120   Positive band

Ladda, R., Atkins, L., Littlefield, J., Neurath, P. and Marimuthu, K. M.: Computer-assisted analysis of chromosomal abnormalities: Detection of a deletion in Aniridia-Wilm's tumor syndrome. Science 185:784-787, 1974.
Patient T. M. (MGH 167-19-15) in this report.
46,XX or XY,ins(8p+;11q-).
46,XX or XY,ins(8;11)(p12p22;q21q24).
46,XX or XY,ins(8;11)(8pter to 8p22::11q24 to 11q21::8p12 or 8p21 to 8qter;11pter to 11q21::11q24 to 11qter).
A segment of 8(:8p12 to 8p22:) appears to have been deleted, i.e., this karyotype shows an unbalanced interstitial translocation with monosomy for a portion of 8p.

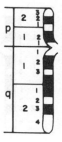

08p210   Negative band

Lubs, H. A. and Lubs, M. L.: New cytogenetic technics applied to a series of children with mental retardation. Nobel Symposium 23:241-250, 1973.
46,XX,t(8;10)(p21;q26).
Patient No. 3 in this report.
46,XX,-8,+der(8)(p21)mat.
46,XX,-8,+der(8)(8qter to 8p21:)mat.

08p220   Positive band

Same entry as in 08p120 (Ladda et al., 1974).

Same entry as in 01q430 (Martinetti and Noel, 1973).

Same entry as in 0Xp120 (Pearson, van der Linden and Hagemeijer, 1974).

08p230   Negative band

Allderdice, P. W.: A large kindred with segregation of pericentric inversion heterozygotes inv(3)(p25q21) and inv(8)(p23q22). Amer. J. Hum. Genet. 26:9A, 1974 and personal communication, 1974.
46,XX,inv(8)(p23q22).
This inversion was found in four individuals in three generations. It is believed to have been inherited from the proband's maternal grandfa-

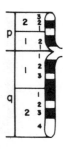

ther. The maternal grandmother is a chromosomal-ly normal member of the inversion 3 kindred. (See Allderdice, 1973 in entry 03p250).

Fujimoto, A. and Wilson, M. G.: Pericentric inversion of chromosome No. 8. Clin. Res. 22:217A., 1974; and Personal Communication from Dr. A. Fujimoto, 1974.
46,XX,inv(8) (p23q22).
46,XX,rec(8),dupq,inv(8) (p23q22).

Jacobs, P. A., Buckton, K. E., Cunningham, C. and Newton, M. S.: An analysis of the break points of structural rearrangements in man. J. Med. Genet. 11:50-64, 1974.
M. R. C. Registry No. K171-214-68 in this report.
46,XX,t(8;18) (p23;p11).
M. R. C. Registry Nos. K4-155-61, K12-92-64, K14-14-65 and K12-77-66 in this report.
46,XX, and XY,inv(8) (p23q11).
46,XX, and XY,inv(8) (pter to p23::q11 to p23::q11 to qter).

Uchida, I. A. and Lin, C. C.: Identification of partial 12 trisomy by quinacrine fluorescence. J. Pediat. 82:269-272, 1973.
46,XY,t(8;12) (p23;p12).
46,XY,t(8;12) (8qter to 8p23::12p12 to 12pter;12q-ter to 12p12::8p2 to 8pter).
46,XX,der(8)t(8;12) (p23;p12)pat.
46,XY,-8,+der(8)t(8;12) (p23;p12)pat.
46,XY,-8,+der(8)t(8;12) (8qter to 8p23::12p12 to 12pter)pat.
Mutant Cell Repository No. GM-213.
See del Solar and Uchida (1974, Case 8 G.S.) in entry 08p000.

08q000

Chen, Y. C. and Woolley, P. V.: Genetic studies on hypospadias in males. J. Med. Genet. 8:153-159, 1971.
47,XXY,t(8;12) (q;q).
Chromosome identification by autoradiography.

Same entry as in 0Xq100 (Cohen et al., 1972).

Same entry as in 03p000 (del Amo and Gullon,

1972).

Same entry as in 02p000 (Handmaker, Hall and Conte, 1974).

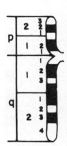

Khudr, G., Naftolin, F., Benirschke, K., Zarate, A. and Guzman-toledano, R.: Unusual transloca- tions and reproductive failure. Obstet. Gynec. 41:542-546, 1973.
46,XX,t(8;13)(q;q3).
46,XX,t(8;13)(8pter to 8q::13q3 to 13qter;13pter to 13q3::8q to 1qter).
46,XX and XY,der(8)der(13)t(8;13)(q;q3)mat.

Leisti, J.: Structural variation in human mitotic chromosomes. Ann. Acad. Sci. fenn, (Med.) Series A, IV, Biologica 179:1-69, 1971.
Case No. 6 in this report.
46,XX,Cq-.

Same entry as in 08+ (Lejeune and Rethore, 1973).

08q100

Same entry as in 0Xq200 (Cohen et al., 1972).

Same entry as in 05p100 (Dutrillaix, 1972).

08q110   Negative band

Same entry as in 08p230 (Jacobs et al., 1974).

08q120   Positive band

Same entry as in 06q270 (Niebuhr, 1973).

08q210   Positive band

Fryns, J. P., Verresen, H., van den Berghe, H., van Kerckvoorde, J. and Cassiman, J. J.: Partial trisomy 8: trisomy of the distal part of the long arm of chromosome number 8+(8q2) in a severely retarded and malformed girl. Humangenetik 24:241-246, 1974.
Case S. A. 030368 in this report.
46,XX,+8q21-24.
46,XX,t(8;13)(q21;p1).
46,XX,t(8;13)(13qter to 13p1::8q21 to 8q24).

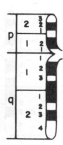

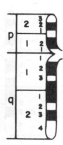

Same entry as in 01q430 (Martinetti and Noel, 1973).

Same entry as in OXp220 (Mikkelsen and Dahl, 1973).

08q220   Negative band

Same entry as in 08p230 (Allderdice, 1974).

Same entry as in 08p230 (Fujimoto and Wilson, 1974).

Lejeune, J., Rethore, M. O., Dutrillaux, B. and Martin, G.: Translocation 8-22 sans changement de longueur et trisomie partielle 8q. Exp. Cell Res. 74:293-295, 1972.
46,XX,t(8;22)(q22;p11).
46,XX,t(8;22)(8pter to 8q22::22p11 to 22pter;22qter to 22p11::8q22 to 8qter).
47,XY,+der(22)t(8;22)(q22;p11)mat.
47,XY,+der(22)t(8;22)(22qter to 22p11::8q22 to 8qter)mat.

Sakurai, M., Oshimura, M., Kakati, S. and Sandberg, A. A.: 8/21 translocation and missing sex chromosomes in acute leukaemia. Lancet 2:227-228, 1974.
46,XX,t(8;21)(q22;q22).
45,X,-Y,t(8;21)(q22;q22).

08q240   Negative band

Same entry as in 08q210 (Fryns et al., 1974).

Same entry as in 02q110 (Worton, 1973).

08q241   Negative band

Sanchez, O. and Yunis, J. J.: Partial trisomy 8 (8q24) and the trisomy-8 syndrome. Humangenetik 23:297-303, 1974.
46,XX,t(8;22)(q241;q11).
Case No. 1 and No. 2 in this report.
47,XX and XY,+der(22)t(8;22)(q241;q11)mat.
47,XX and XY,+der(22)t(8;22)(22pter to 22q11::8q241 to 8qter)mat.

090000

Baccichetti, C. and Tenconi, R.: A new case of trisomy for the short arm of Nc. 9 chromosome. J. Med. Genet. 10:296-299, 1973.
46,XY,-15,+t(9p15q).

Battaglia, E., Guanti, G., Barsanti, P. and Petrinelli, P.: Chromosomal survey in 298 normal subjects and 1,253 cases of congenital disorders during 1966-1970. Acta Genet. Med. Gemellol. 20:123-173, 1971.
46,XY,t(9q12q),t(9p12p).

Centerwall, W. R., Wyatt, J. F., Beatty-DeSana, J. W. and Hoggard, M. J.: Rethore's syndrome. Trisomy of the short arm of chromosome 9. Newport Beach, Calif., Birth Defects Conf., National Foundation - March of Dimes, p. 111, June 16-21, 1974.
46,XY,-14,+t(9p14q).

Craig-Holmes, A. P., Moore, F. B. and Shaw, M. W.: Polymorphism of human C-band heterochromatin. I. Frequency of variants. Amer. J. Hum. Genet. 25:181-192, 1973.

Same entry as in 0X0000 (Dumars and Reed, 1974).

Leisti, J.: Structural variation in human mitotic chromosomes. Ann. Acad. Sci. fenn. (Med.) Series A, IV, Biologica 179:1-69, 1971. Case No. 13 in this report.
46,XY,r(9).

Martin, A. O., Turk, K. B. and Macintyre, M. N.: An analysis of chromosome 9 inversions in four families. Amer. J. Hum. Genet. 26:58A, 1974.
46,XX,inv(9)/47,XX,inv(9),+inv(9).

09p000

Same entry as in 04q000 (Buckton, 1972).

Dinno, N. D., Silvey, G. L. and Weisskopf, B.: 47,XY,t(9p+;11q+) in a male infant with multiple malformations. Clin. Genet. 6:125-131, 1974. Patient E.C. in this report.

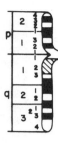

47,XY,+t(9p+;11q+).
"Fluorescence microscopy revealed that the extra
chromosome was aberrant. The short arms were
those of chromosome number 9 and the long arms
those of chromosome number 11...".

Ebbin, A. J., Wilson, M. G., Towner, J. W. and
Slaughter, J. P.: Prenatal diagnosis of an
inherited translocation between chromosomes No. 9
and 18. J. Med. Genet. 10:65-69, 1973.
46,XX,t(9;18)(p;p11).
46,XX,-18,+der(18)t(9;18)(p;p11)mat.
46,XX,-18,+der(18)t(9;18)(18qter to 18p11::9p to
9pter)mat.

Same entry as in 05q000 (Fredga and Hall, 1970).

Guanti, G., Battaglia, E., Petrinelli, P. and
Rigillo, N.: A family with a balanced C/C
translocation carrier and an unbalanced
47,XY,(Cq-)+ son. Acta Genet. Med. Gemellol.
20:245-255, 1971.
46,XY,t(9;12)(p;q1).
47,XY,+der(12)t(9;12)(p;q1)pat.

Howard, P. N., Stoddard, G. R. and Seely, J. R.:
Giemsa banding of a human metacentric chromosome
number 9. Humangenetik 18:271-272, 1973.
46,XX,inv(9)(pq).

Jacobsen, P., Mikkelsen, M. and Rosleff, F.: A
ring chromosome, diagnosed by quinacrine fluorescence as No. 9, in a mentally retarded girl.
Clin. Genet. 4:434-441, 1973.
46,XX,r(9).

Kistenmacher, M. L. and Punnett, H. H.: Compara-
tive behavior of ring chromosomes. Amer. J. Hum.
Genet. 22:304-318, 1970.
Case I (J.S. SCHC No. 6700059) in this report.
46,XY,r(9)(pq).
Mutant Cell Repository No. GM-166.

Leisti, J.: Structural variation in human
mitotic chromosomes. Ann. Acad. Sci. fenn.
(Med.) Series A, IV, Biologica 179:1-69, 1971.
Case No. 5 in this report.
46,XX,9p-.

Case No. 22 in this report.
46,XY,9p+.

Lubs, H. A. and Ruddle, F. H.: Chromosome polymorphism in American Negro and White populations. Nature 233:134-136, 1971.
inv(9)(pq).

Madan, K. and Bobrow, M.: Structural variation in chromosome no. 9. Ann. Genet. 17:81-86, 1974.
46,XX and XY,inv(9)(pq).

Weber, F. M., Muller, H. and Sparkes, R. S.: The 9p+ syndrome due to inherited translocation. Newport Beach, Calif., Birth Defects Conf., National Foundation - March of Dimes, p. 86, June 16-21, 1974.
46,XY,t(9;22)(p;p1).
46,XX,-22,+der(22)t(9;22)(p;p1)pat.
46,XX,-22,+der(22)t(9;22)(22qter to 22p1::9p to 9pter)pat.

09p100

de la Chapelle, A.: Personal Communication, 1974 and Rotterdam Conference, 1974.
46,XY,inv(9)(p1q13).
Meiosis was found to be normal in male carriers of this variant chromosome. Inversion homozygotes were also found in this kindred.
46,XY,inv(9)(p1q13).
Mutant Cell Repository No. GM-445.
Mutant Cell Repository No. GM-447.
Mutant Cell Repository No. GM-450.
46,XX,inv(9)(p1q13).
Mutant Cell Repository No. GM-453.

Lejeune, J.: Scientific impact of the study of fine structure of chromatids. Nobel Symposium 23:16-24, 1973.
See Rethore et al. (1970) in entry 09p100.

Lejeune, J., Berger, R., Rethore, M. O., Salmon, C. and Kaplan, M.: Translocation Cc-F familiale, determinant une trisomie pour le bras court du chromosome 12. Ann. Genet. 9:12-18, 1966.

Rethore, M. O., Larget-Piet, L., Abonyi, D.,

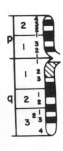

Boeswillwald, M., Berger, R., Carpentier, S., Cruveiller, J., Dutrillaux, B., Lafourcade, J., Penneau, M. and Lejeune, J.: Sur quatre cas de trisomie pour le bras court due chromosome 9. Individualisation d'une nouvelle entite morbide. Ann. Genet. 13:217-232, 1970.
46,XX,t(9;19) (p1;p13).
46,XX,t(9;19) (9qter to 9p1::19p13 to 19pter;19qter to 19p13::9p1 to 9pter).
Case No. IP 1493 in this report.
46,XY,-19,+der(19)t(9;19) (p1;p13)mat.
46,XY,-19,+der(19)t(9;19) (19qter to 19p13::9p1 to 9pter)mat.
46,XY,t(9;22) (p1;p1).
46,XY,t(9;22) (9qter to 9p1::22p1 to 22pter;22qter to 22p1::9p1 to 9pter.
Case IP 5340 in this report.
46,XX and XY,-22,+der(22)t(9;22) (p1;p1)pat.
46,XX and XY,-22,+der(22)t(9;22) (22qter to 22p1::9p1 to 9pter)pat.
Additional information was obtained from the article by Lejeune (1973) cited in entry 09p100.

Wahrman, J., Atidia, J., Goitein, R. and Cohen, T.: Pericentric inversions of chromosome 9 in two families. Cytogenetics 11:132-144, 1972.
46,XX and XY,inv(9) (p1q1).
Chromosome identification by autoradiography.

09p110   Negative band

Same entry as in 01q440 (Dewald, Spurbeck and Gordon, 1974).

Jacobs, P. A., Melville, M. and Ratcliffe, S.: A cytogenetic survey of 11,680 newborn infants. Ann. Hum. Genet. 37:359-374, 1974.
M. R. C. Registry No. 192-72 in this report.
46,XX,inv(9) (p11q13).
46,XX,inv(9) (pter to p11::q13 to p11::q13 to qter).
M. R. C. Registry No. 226-72 in this report.
46,XX,inv(9) (p11q12).
46,XX,inv(9) (pter to p11::q12 to p11::q12 to qter).

09p130   Negative band

Lin, C. C., Holman, G. and Sewell, L.: Inherited translocation t(9;11)(p13;p15) and partial trisomy 9p syndrome. Amer. J. Hum. Genet. 26:54A, 1974.
46,XX,t(9;11)(p13;p15).
This mother had 10 children, three of whom have a partial duplication of the short arm of chromosome No. 9 and a partial deletion of the short arm of chromosome No. 11.

09p200

Alfi, O. S., Donnell, G. N., Crandall, B. F., Derencsenyi, A. and Menon, R.: Deletion of the short arm of chromosome #9 (46,9p-): A new deletion syndrome. Ann. Genet. 16:17-22, 1973.
46,XX,t(9;16)(p2;q2).
46,XX,der(9)der(16)t(9;16)(p2;q2)mat.
Patient No. 1 in this report.
46,XX,-9,+der(9)t(9;16)(p2q2)mat.
Patient No. 2 in this report.
46,XY,del(9)(p2).
46,XY,del(9)(qter to p2:).

Same entry as in 0Xq100 (Cohen et al., 1972).

Francke, U.: Quinacrine mustard fluorescence of human chromosomes: characterization of unusual translocations. Amer. J. Hum. Genet. 24:189-213, 1972.
46,XX,t(9;18)(p2;q).
Case 8: SD 030170 in this report.
47,XX,+der(18)t(9;18)(p2;q)mat.

Same entry as in 04q280 (Jacobs et al., 1974).

Rethore, M. O., Dutrillaux, B., Baheux, G., Gerveaux, C. and Lejeune, J.: Monosomie pour les regions juxtacentromeriques d'un chromosome 21. Exp. Cell Res. 70:455-456, 1972.
45,XX,-9,-21,+t(9;21)(p2;q2).
45,XX,-9,-21,+t(9;21)(9qter to 9p2::21q2 to 21qter).

Short, E. M., Solitaire, G. B. and Breg, W. R.: A case of partial 14 trisomy 47,XX,(14q-)+ and translocation t(9p+;14q-) in mother and brother. J. Med. Genet. 9:367-373, 1972.

46,XX,t(9;14)(p2;q2).
46,XY,der(9)der(14)t(9;14)(p2q2)mat.
47,XY,+der(14)t(9;14)(p2;q2)mat.

09p210   Positive band

Same entry as in 01q430 (Martinetti and Noel, 1973).

09p220   Negative band

Hamerton, J. L., Ray, M. and Douglas, G. R.: Chromosome banding techniques in clinical cytogenetics. Nobel Symposium 23:209-213, 1973.
46,XX,t(9;18)(p22;q21).
46,XX,t(9;18)(9qter to 9p22::18q21 to 18qter;18pter to 18q21::9p22 to 9pter).
Case III: D110472, NB-8762 in this report.
46,XY,-18,+der(18)t(9;18)(p22;q21)mat.
46,XY,-18,+der(18)t(9;18)(18pter to 18q21::9p22 to 9pter)mat.

Same entry as in 03q210 (Kreiger, Palmer and Biegel, 1974).

09p240   Negative band

Buckton, K. E.: The identification of whole chromosomes or parts of chromosomes by the new banding techniques. Nobel Symposium 23:196-200, 1972.
46,XY,t(9;16)(p24;q11).
46,XX,-9,+der(9)t(9;16)(p24;q11)pat.

Same entry as in 02q330 (Rosenthal et al., 1974).

Sekhon, G. S. and Kaufman, R. L.: Centromeric suppression or two functional centromeres in a stable dicentric? Amer. J. Hum. Genet. 26:77A, 1974.
45,XX or XY,-9,-11+.
t(9;11)(p24:p15).
End to end fusion is hypothesized with inactivation or suppression of centromere of chromosome 9.

Same entry as in 0Xq120 (Shows and Brown, 1974).

09q000

Same entry as in 01p000 (Buckton, 1972).

Same entry as in 03p000 (del Amo et al., 1971, Case MA 261066).

Dumars, K. W., Reed, P. and Lawce, H.: Autosome X translocation in a family with a marker Y chromosome. Amer. J. Hum. Genet. 26:27A, 1974.
Patient BR 121263 in this report.
47,XYqs,t(Xq+;9p-).
The satellited Y chromosome is apparently the same as that reported by Genest (1973) in 0Yq100.

Same entry as in 09p000 (Howard, Stoddard and Seely, 1973).

Leisti, J.: Structural variation in human mitotic chromosomes. Ann. Acad. Sci. fenn. (Med.) Series A, IV, Biologica 179:1-69, 1971.
46,XX,t(9q+;Dq-).
Case No. 16 in this report.
45,XX,-9,-D,+der(9)t(9q+;Dq-)mat.

Newton, M. S., Cunningham, C., Jacobs, P. A., Price, W. H. and Fraser, I. A.: Chromosome survey of a hospital for the mentally subnormal. Part 2: Autosome abnormalities. Clin. Genet. 3:226-248, 1972.
46,XX,t(9q-;22p+).
M. R. C. Registry No. K68-178-69 in this report.
47,XY,+der(9)t(9q-;22p+)mat.

Rary, J. M., Park, I. J., Heller, R. H., Jones, H. W. and Baramki, T. A.: Prenatal cytogenetic analyses of women with high risk for genetic disorders. J. Hered. 65:209-212, 1974.
46,XX,t(9q+;13q-).
47,X?,der(13)t(9q+;13q-).
This child was previously thought to be trisomy 21 and died at the age of six months. 'A closer examination of the medical records.....indicated to us that the child was perhaps not a trisomy 21 but in all probability did possess an unbalanced set of chromosomes arising from the translocation in the mother.'
See also Rary (1974) in entry 09q220.

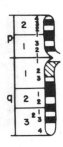

Sarto, G. E.: Cytogenetics of fifty patients
with primary amenorrhea. Amer. J. Obstet. Gynec.
119:14-23, 1974.
46,XX,t(9q-;10q+).

Schmid, W.: The prenatal diagnosis of chromosome
anomalies. Triangle 11:91-102, 1972.
46,XX,t(9q-;18q+).
46,XX and XY,der(9)der(18)t(9q-;18q+)mat.

09q100

Evans, H. J., Buckton, K. E. and Sumner, A. T.:
Cytological mapping of human chromosomes: Results
obtained with quinacrine fluorescence and the
acetic-saline-Giemsa techniques. Chromosoma
34:448-454, 1971.
46,XX,t(9;22)(q1;p1).
46,XY,der(9)der(22)t(9;22)(q1;p1)mat.
47,XY,+der(9)t(9;22)(q1;p1)mat.
See Buckton (1972) in entry 09q120.

Lejeune, J.: Scientific impact of the study of
fine structure of chromatids. Nobel Symposium
23:16-24, 1973.
See Rethore et al. (1970) in entry 09q100.

Rethore, M. O., Larget-Piet, L., Abonyi, D.,
Boeswillwald, M., Berger, R., Carpentier, S.,
Cruveiller, J., Dutrillaux, B., Lafourcade, J.,
Penneau, M. and Lejeune, J.: Sur quatre cas de
trisomie pour le bras court du chromosome 9.
Individualisation d'une nouvelle entite morbide.
Ann. Genet. 13:217-232, 1970.
46,XX,t(9;22)(q1;q13).
46,XX,t(9;22)(9pter to 9q1::22q13 to 22qter;22p-
ter to 22q13::9q1 to 9qter).
Case No. 2 in this report.
47,XX,+der(9)t(9;22)(q1;q13)mat.
47,XX,+der(9)t(9;22)(9pter to 9q1::22q13 to
22qter)mat.
Additional information was obtained from the
article by Lejeune (1973) cited in entry 09q100.

Smith, G. F., Sachdeva, S. and Justice, P.: A
chromosomal break and partial deletion of a
number 9 chromosome. Hum. Hered. 23:561-567,
1974.

46,XY,del(9)(q).
46,XY,del(9)(pter to q:).
"Chromosomal studies revealed that the child was
mosaic for a chromosomal fragment from the long
arms of a number 9 chromosome. The majority of
cells contained 46 chromosomes with a partially
deleted number 9 chromosome and a chromosomal
fragment."

Same entry as in 09p100 (Wahrman et al., 1972).

09q110   Negative band

Same entry as in 01q440 (Kreiger, Palmer and
Biegel, 1974).

09q120   Variable band

Same entry as in 04q300 (Bobrow, Madan and
Pearson, 1972).

Buckton, K. E.: The identification of whole
chromosomes or parts of chromosomes by the new
banding techniques. Nobel Symposium 23:196-200,
1972.
46,XX,t(9;22)(q12;p1).
47,XY,+der(9)t(9;22)(q12;p1)mat.
See Evans, Buckton and Sumner (1971) in entry
09q100 and Chandley et al. (1972) in entry
09q120.

Chandley, A. C., Christie, S., Fletcher, J. M.,
Frackiewicz, A. and Jacobs, P. A.: Translocation
heterozygosity and associated subfertility in
man. Cytogenetics 11:516-533, 1972.
46,XX,t(9;22)(q12;p1).
46,XX,t(9;22)(9pter to 9q12::22p1 to 22pter;22q-
ter to 22p1::9q12 to 9qter).
M. R. C. Registry Nos. K68-32-70 and K68-149-70
in this report.
46,XY,der(9)der(22)t(9;22)(q12;p1)mat.
Seminal analysis indicated azoospermia.
M. R. C. Registry No. K68-178-69 in this report.
47,XY,+der(9)t(9;22)(q12;p1)mat.
47,XY,+der(9)t(9;22)(9pter to 9q12::22p1 to
22pter)mat.

Fitzgerald, P. H.: The nature and inheritance of

an elongated secondary constriction on chromosome 9 of man. Cytogenet. Cell Genet. 12:404-413, 1973.
46,XX and XY,9qh+.
The variant chromosome was detected in 17 individuals belonging to three generations of a family. There were twice as many carriers as non-carriers suggesting disturbed segregation which is presumed to be consistent with the increased heterochromatin present.

Same entry as in 09p110 (Jacobs, Melville and Ratcliffe, 1974).

Same entry as in 06p250 (Rethore et al., 1970).

Madan, K. and Bobrow, M.: Structural variation in chromosome no. 9. Ann. Genet 17:81-86, 1974.
46,XX and XY,9qh+.

Mikelsaar, A. V. N., Tuur, S. J. and Kyaosaar, M. E.: Human karyotype polymorphism. I. Routine and fluorescence microscopic investigation of chromosomes in a normal adult population. Humangenetik 20:89-101, 1973.
46,XX and XY,9qh+.

Nielsen, J., Friedrich, U., Hreidarsson, A. B. and Zeuthen, E.: Frequency of 9qh+ and risk of chromosome aberrations in the progeny of individuals with 9qh+. Humangenetik 21:211-216, 1974.
The authors concluded that 9qh+ probably represents a duplication and it was present with a 0.1% frequency in the five populations studied. The individuals possessing the variant have an increased risk of chromosome abnormalities in the progeny.

Palmer, C. G. and Schroder, J.: A familial variant of chromosome 9. J. Med. Genet. 8:202-207, 1971.

09q130   Negative band

Same entry as in 09p100 (de la Chapelle, 1974).

Same entry as in 09p110 (Jacobs, Melville and Ratcliffe, 1974).

09q210   Positive band

Buckton, K. E.:   The identification of whole chromosomes or parts of chromosomes by the new banding techniques. Nobel Symposium 23:196-200, 1972.
46,XX,t(9;22)(q21;q11).
46,XY,-22,+der(22)t(9;22)(q21;q11)mat.

Friedrich, U. and Nielsen, J.:   Autosomal reciprocal translocations in newborn children and their relatives. Humangenetik 21:133-144, 1974.
46,XY,t(9;19)(q21;q13).
46,XY,t(9;19)(9pter to 9q21::19q13 to 19qter;19pter to 19q13::9q21 to 9qter).
46,XX and XY,der(9)der(19)t(9;19)(q21;q13)mat and pat.
Proband Nos. 2525 and 9273 in this report.
46,XX and XY,der(9)der(19)t(9;19)(q21;q13)pat.

Hirschhorn, K., Lucas, M. and Wallace, I.: Precise identification of various chromosomal abnormalities.   Ann. Hum. Genet. 36:375-379, 1973.
Family A(Gc 759) in this report.
46,XY,t(9;22)(q21;q11).
46,XX,-22,+der(22)t(9;22)(q21;q11)pat.
46,XX,-22,+der(22)t(9;22)(22pter to 22q11::9q21 to 9qter)pat.

09q220   Negative band

Howard, P. N., Yarbrough, K. M. and Stoddard, G. R.:   C9/D13/translocation resulting in duplication deficiency.   Newport Beach, Calif., Birth Defects Conf., National Foundation - March of Dimes, p. 132, June 16-21, 1974.
46,XX,t(9;13)(q22;q12).
46,XX,t(9;13)(9pter to 9q22::13q12 to 13qter;13pter to 13q12::9q22 to 9qter).
46,XX,-13,+der(9)t(9;13)(q22;q12)mat.
46,XX,-13,+der(9)t(9;13)(9pter to 9q22::13q12 to 13qter)mat.
47,XX or XY,+der(13)rcp(9;13)(q22;q14)mat.

Same entry as in 01p320 (Jacobs et al., 1974).

Rary, J. M.:   Personal Communication, 1974.

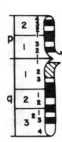

Case No. 47 in this laboratory.
46,XX,rcp(9;13)(q22;q14).
See Rary et al. (1974) in entry 09q000.

09q300

Haeffler, G. and Hall, B.: A dysplastic girl
with an inherited partial C trisomy. Acta
Obstet. Gynec. Scand. 49:311-314, 1970.
46,XX,t(?9;?11)(q3;q1).
46,XY,der(?9)der(?11)t(?9;?11)(q3;q1)mat.
46,XX,-11,+der(?11)t(?9;?11)(q3;q1)mat.
Chromosome identification by morphology.

Same entry as in 06q100 (Rohde and Catz, 1964).

Same entry as in 22q100 (Rowley, 1973).

09q320   Negative band

Same entry as in 0Xq110 (Leisti, 1974).

09q330   Positive band

Aula, P. and Karjalainen, O.: Prenatal karyotype
analysis in high risk families. Ann. Clin. Res.
5:142-148, 1973.
46,XX,t(9;15)(q33;q12).
46,XX,t(9;15)(9pter to 9q33::15q12 to 15qter;15p-
ter to 15q12::9q33 to 9qter).
Case No. 7 in this report.
45,XX,-9,-15,+der(9)t(9;15)(q33;q12)mat.
45,XX,-9,-15,+der(9)t(9;15)(9pter to q33::15q12
to 15qter)mat.
Fetal material was karyotyped.

09q340   Negative band

Danilowicz, D. A., Feingold, M. and Wolman, S.:
Polyvalvular mucopolysaccharidosis of the heart
in an infant with C/D chromosomal translocation.
Amer. J. Cardiol. 32:105-109, 1973.
45,XX,t(9;14)(q34;q11).
45,XX,t(9;14)(9pter to 9q34::14q11 to 14qter).

Whang-Peng, J., Lee, E. C. and Knutsen, T. A.:
Genesis of the Ph1 chromosome. J. Nat. Cancer
Inst. 52:1035-1036, 1974.

46,XX and XY,t(9;22)(q34:q12).
Chromosome identification done by Giemsa banding
technique in a patient with chronic myeloid
leukemia.

Same entry as in 02q210 (Weitkamp, 1974).

100000

Lewandowsky, R., Sanchez, O. and Yunis, J. J.: A
new syndrome resulting from partial trisomy for
the distal third of the long arm of chromosome
10. Amer. J. Hum. Genet. 26:53A, 1974.

Same entry as in 06q210 (Thurmon, Robertson and
Campbell, 1974).

10p100

Atkins, L., Pant, S. S., Hazard, G. W. and
Ouellette, E. M.: Two cases with a C group ring.
Ann. Hum. Genet. 30:1-6, 1966.
46,XY,r(?10).

Elliott, D., Thomas, G. H., Condron, C. J.,
Khuri, N. and Richardson, F.: C-group chromosome
abnormality (?10p-). Amer. J. Dis. Child.
119:72-73, 1970.
46,XX,?del(10)(p1).
46,XX,?del(10)(qter to p1:).

10p110   Negative band

de la Chapelle, A.: Personal Communication,
1974.
46,XY,inv(10)(p11q11).
Mutant Cell Repository No. GM-445.
46,XY,inv(10)(p11q21).
Mutant Cell Repository No. GM-445.
Mutant Cell Repository No. GM-452.

Same entry as in 07p220 (Schleiermacher et al.,
1974).

10p130   Negative band

Francke, U., Mahan, G. M., Dixson, B. K. and
Jones, O. W.: New autosomal deletion syndrome:

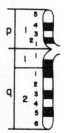

10p-.   Newport Beach, Calif., Birth Defects
Conf., National Foundation - March of Dimes, p.
87, June 16-21, 1974.
46,XX,del(10)(p13).
46,XX,del(10)(qter to p13:).

10p150   Negative band

Dutrillaux, B., Laurent, C., Robert, J. M. and
Lejeune, J.: Pericentric inversion, inv(10), in
a mother and aneusomy by recombination, inv
(10),rec(10), in her son.   Cytogenet. Cell
Genet. 12:245-253, 1973.
46,XX,inv(10)(p15q24).
46,XX,inv(10)(pter to p15::q24 to p15::q24 to
qter).
46,XY,rec(10)(qter to q24::p15 to qter).

10q000

Same entry as in 02q000 (Buckton, 1972).

del Solar, C. and Uchida, I. A.: Identification
of chromosomal abnormalities by quinacrine-
staining technique in patients with normal
karyotypes by conventional analysis. J. Pediat.
84:534-538, 1974.
Case No. 17, T. B. in this report.
46,XX,10q+

Dutrillaux, B.:   Nouveau systeme de marquage
chromosomique: Les bandes T. Chromosoma 41:395-
402, 1973.
t(10q-;18q+).

Same entry as in 05p100 (Ferguson-Smith, 1972).
Since that paper was submitted, mitotic analysis
by Giemsa banding showed that the chromosome
involved was #10 and not #8.

Same entry as in 05p100 (Lubs and Lubs, 1974).

Same entry as in 04q000 (Newton et al., 1972).

Same entry as in 09q000 (Sarto, 1974).

Sarto, G. E.:   Cytogenetics of fifty patients
with primary amenorrhea. Amer. J. Obstet. Gynec.

119:14-23, 1974.
46,XX,t(10q+;12q-).

10q110   Negative band

Same entry as in 10p110 (de la Chapelle, 1974).

Same entry as in 05q330 (Hirschhorn, Lucas and Wallace, 1973).

Hirschhorn, K., Lucas, M. and Wallace, I.: Precise identification of various chromosomal abnormalities. Ann. Hum. Genet. 36:375-379, 1973.
Family Le(Gc 628) in this report.
46,XX,t(10;15)(q11;q24).
46,XX,t(10;15)(10pter to 10q11::15q24 to 15qter;15pter to 15q24::10q11 to 10qter).

Same entry as in 05q330 (Lucas and Wallace, 1972).

Same entry as in 07p200 (Miller, Coriell and Greene, 1974).

10q200

Francke, U.: Quinacrine mustard fluorescence of human chromosomes: characterization of unusual translocations. Amer. J. Hum. Genet. 24:189-213, 1972.
Case No. 2: LS 020951 in this report.
46,XX,t(10;22)(q2;p1),21q+.
46,XX,t(10;15)(q2;p1).
Case No. 6: KW 061268 in this report.
46,XX,-15,+der(15)t(10;15)(q2;p1)mat.
46,XX,-15,+der(15)t(10;15)(15qter to 15p1::10q2 to 10qter)mat.

Same entry as in 04q000 (Jacobs et al., 1974).

Talvik, T. A., Mikelsaar, A. V. N., Mikelsaar, R., Kyaosaar, M. E., and Tuur, S. J.: Inherited translocations in two families [t(14q+;10q-)] and t(13q-;21q+). Humangenetik 19:215-226, 1973.
Family F1 in this report.
46,XY,t(10;14)(q2;q3).
46,XY,t(10;14)(10pter to 10q2::14q3 to

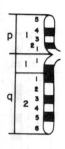

14qter;14pter to 14q3::10q2 to 10qter).
46,XX and XY,-14,+der(14)t(10;14)(q2;q3)pat.
46,XX and XY,-14,+der(14)t(10;14)(14pter to
14q3::10q2 to 10qter)pat.
This patient is partially monosomic for the long
arm of chromosome No. 14 and partially trisomic
for the long arm of chromosome 10.

Yunis, J. J. and Sanchez, O.: A new syndrome
resulting from partial trisomy for the distal
third of the long arm of chromosome 10. J.
Pediat. 84:567-570, 1974.
46,XX,t(10;15)(q2;q26).
46,XY,der(10)der(15)t(10;15)(q2;q26)mat.
46,XY,-15,+der(15)t(10;15)(q2;q26)pat.
46,XY,-15,+der(15)t(10;15)(15pter to 15q26::10q2
to 10qter)pat.

10q210   Positive band

Same entry as in 10p110 (de la Chapelle, 1974).

10q220   Negative band

Same entry as in 05q350 (Boue and Boue, 1973).

Same entry as in 03q280 (Friedrich and Nielsen,
1974).

Same entry as in 02q110 (Jacobs et al., 1974).

Same entry as in 01q440 (Laurent, Bovier-Lapierre
and Dutrillaux, 1973).

10q230   Positive band

Same entry as in 04q350 (Buckton, 1972).

Ferguson-Smith, M. A. and Page, B. M.: Pachytene
analysis in a human reciprocal (10;11) translocation. J. Med. Genet. 10:282-287, 1973.
46,XY,t(10;11)(q23;q24).
46,XY,t(10;11)(10pter to 10q23::11q24 to
11qter;11pter to 11q24::10q23 to 10qter).
MI,22,XY,IV(10;11) or MI,23,X,Y,IV(10;11).
46,XX,-11,+der(11)t(10;11)(q23;q24)pat.
46,XX,-11,+der(11)t(10;11)(11pter to 11q24::10q23
to 10qter)pat.

10q240   Negative band

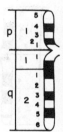

Boue, J. and Boue, A.: L'interet en diagnostic
prenatal des techniques nouvelle d'identification
chromosomique dans des translocations et une
aneusome de recombinaison.   Nouv. Presse Med.
2:3097-3102, 1973.
Observation LA95 in this report.
46,XX,t(10;22)(q24;p12).
46,XX,t(10;22)(10pter to 10q24::22p12 to
22pter;22qter to 22p12::10q24 to 10qter).

Same entry as in 10p150 (Dutrillaux et al.,
1973).

Mellman, W. J.: Personal Communication, 1974.
46,XY,t(10;17)(q24;p13).
Mutant Cell Repository No. GM-215.
46,XX,der(17)t(10;17)(q24;p13)pat.
Mutant Cell Repository No. GM-217.

Roux, C., Taillemite, J. L. and Baheux-Morlier,
G.: Partial trisomy 10q due to a familial t(10q-
;22p+). Ann. Genet. 17:59-62, 1974.
46,XX and XY,t(10;22)(q24;p12).
46,XX and XY,t(10;22)(10pter to 10q24::22p12 to
22pter;22qter to 22p12::10q24 to 10qter).
46,XY,-22,+der(22)t(10;22)(q24;p12)mat.
46,XY,-22,+der(22)t(10;22)(22qter to 22p12::10q24
to 10qter)mat.

10q260   Negative band

Same entry as in 08p210 (Lubs and Lubs, 1973).

110000

Breg, W. R., Miller, D. A., Allderdice, P. W. and
Miller, O. J.: Identification of translocation
chromosomes by quinacrine fluorescence. Amer. J.
Dis. Child. 123:561-564, 1972.
46,XX,t(11p17q)t(11q17p).
Patient No. 5 in this report.
46,XY,der(11)der(17)t(11p17q)t(11q17p)mat.
46,XX,der(11)der(17)t(11p17q)t(11q17p)mat,del(18)
(q1).

11p100

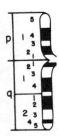

Same entry as in 02p100 (Breg et al., 1972).

de la Chapelle, A.:   Rotterdam Conference, 1974.
inv(11)(pq).

Same entry as in 02q300 (Falk et al., 1973).

Francke,   U.:   Quinacrine mustard fluorescence of
human   chromosomes: characterization   of   unusual
translocations.   Amer. J. Hum. Genet. 24:189-213,
1972.
Case 4: LL 100668 in this report.
46,XX,t(11;17)(p1;q2).

Same entry as in 02q300 (Francke, 1972).

11p110   Negative band

Same entry as in 010000 (Thompson, 1974).

11p120   Positive band

Sanchez,   O.,   Yunis,   J.   J. and Escobar, J. I.:
Partial   trisomy   11   in a child resulting from a
complex maternal rearrangement of chromosomes 11,
12 and 13.   Humangenetik 22:59-65, 1974.
46,XX,t(11;12;13)(p12p15q141q23;p11q241;q34).
46,XX,t(11;12;13)(11pter   to   11p15::11q141   to
11q23::11p11   to   11q13::11q24 to 11qter;12pter to
12p11::11p14   to   11p12::12p11 to 12q23::13q34 to
13qter;13pter to 13q33::12q241 to 12qter).
46,XX,-12,-13,+der(12)+
der(13)t(11;12;13)(p12p15q141q23;p11q241;q34)mat.
46,XX,-12,-13,+der(12)+der(13)t(11;12;13)(12pter
to   12p11::11p14   to   11p12::12p11 to 12q23::13q34
to 13qter;13pter to 13q33::12q241 to 12qter)mat.
Giemsa   banding technique was used to analyze the
chromosomes from early metaphases to identify the
sub-bands in this interesting case.

11p150   Negative band

Francke, U.:   Rotterdam Conference, 1974.
t(11;17)(p15;q21).
See other reference.

Francke, U.:   Regional mapping of human MDH-1 and
IDH-1   on   chromosome   2, LDH-A on chromosome 11,

and thymidine kinase on chromosome 17. Amer. J. Hum. Genet. 26:31A, 1974.
46,XX,t(11;17)(p15;q13).

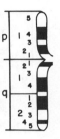

Jacobs, P. A., Buckton, K. E., Cunningham, C. and Newton, M. S.: An analysis of the break points of structural rearrangements in man. J. Med. Genet. 11:50-64, 1974.
M. R. C. Registry No. K203-146-72 in this report.
46,XX,t(11;17)(p15;q11).

Same entry as in 05p110 (Jacobs et al., 1974).

Same entry as in 09p130 (Lin, Holman and Sewell, 1974).

McAlpine, P. J., Chudley, A. E., Bauder, F., Ray, M. and Hamerton, J. L.: Exclusion of peptidase-A structural gene locus from the q11q21 region of chromosome 18 in man. Birth Defects: Original Article Series X(3):126-127, 1974.
46,XY,ins(11;18)(p15;q11q21).
46,XY,ins(11;18)(11pter to 11p15::18q11 to 18q21::11p15 to 11qter;18pter to 18q11::18q21 to 18qter).
46,XX and XY,-18,+der(18)ins
(11;18)(p15;q11q21)pat.
46,XX and XY,-18,+der(18)ins(11;18)(18pter to 18q11::18q21 to 18qter).

Same entry as in 11p120 (Sanchez, Yunis and Escobar, 1974).

Same entry as in 09p240 (Sekton and Kaufman, 1974).

11q000

Bochkov, N. P., Kuleshov, N. P., Chebotarev, A. N., Alekhin, V. I. and Midian, S. A.: Population cytogenetic investigation of newborns in Moscow. Humangenetik 22:139-152, 1974.
46,XY,t(11q-;15q-).

Breg, W. R., Schreck, R. R. and Miller, O. J.: Familial partial trisomy 15: identification of a deleted No. 15 confirmed by anti-5-methylcytodine antibody binding. Amer. J. Hum. Genet. 26:17A,

1974.
46,XX,t(11q+;15q-).
47,XX and XY,der t(15q-)mat.

Same entry as in 11p100 (de la Chapelle, 1974).

Same entry as in 09p000 (Dinno, Silvey and Weisskopf, 1974).

Same entry as in 04q300 (Francke, 1972).

Same entry as in 05q000 (Lubs and Lubs, 1974).

Same entry as in 06p000 (Wright, Clark and Breg, 1974).

11q 100

Same entry as in 09q300 (Haeffler and Hall, 1970).

Same entry as in 07q000 (Leisti, 1971).

Same entry as in 05p100 (Mann and Rafferty, 1972).

Nakagome, Y., Iinuma, K. and Matsui, I.: Three translocations involving C- or G-group chromosomes. J. Med. Genet. 10:174-176, 1973.
Case B in this report.
46,XX,t(11;14)(q12 or 13;q32?).
46,XX,t(11;14)(11pter to 11q12 or 13::14q32? to 14qter;14pter to 14q32?::11q12 or 13 to 11qter).

Rott, M. D., Schwanitz, G., Grosse, K. P. and Alexandrow, G.: C11-D13 translocation in four generations. Humangenetik 14:300-305, 1972.
46,XY,t(11;13)(q1;q3).
46,XX and XY,der(11)der(13)t(11;13)(q1;q3)mat and pat.
47,XXX,der(11)der(13)t(11;13)(q1;q13)pat.
46,XX and XY,-13,+der(13)t(11;13)(q1;q3)pat.
46,XX and XY,-13,+der(13)t(11;13)(13pter to 13q3::11q1 to 11qter)pat.
In this family two children had partial trisomy for the long arm of chromosome 11.

11q130   Negative band

Hamerton, J. L., Ray, M. and Douglas, G. R.:
Chromosome banding techniques in clinical cytogenetics. Nobel Symposium 12:209-213, 1973.
Case II: H070672 NB-9351 in this report.
46,XX,t(11;20)(q13;p13).
46,XX,t(11;20)(11pter to 11q13::20p13 to
20pter;20qter to 20p13::11q13 to 11qter).

Same entry as in 01q210 (Jacobs et al., 1974).

Jacobs, P. A., Buckton, K. E., Cunningham, C. and
Newton, M. S.: An analysis of the break points
of structural rearrangements in man. J. Med.
Genet. 11:50-64, 1974a.
M. R. C. Registry Nos. K72-22-70 and K72-178-71
in this report.
46,XX and XY,t(11;13)(q13;q21).
The two individuals are sibs.
See Jacobs et al. (1974b) in entry 11q130.

Jacobs, P. A., Melville, M., Ratcliffe, S., Keay,
A. J. and Syme, J.: A cytogenetic survey of
11,680 newborn infants. Ann. Hum. Genet. 37:359-
376, 1974b.
M. R. C. Registry Nos. 178-71 and 22-70 in this
report.
46,XX and XY,t(11;13)(q13;q21).
See Jacobs et al. (1974a) in entry 11q130.

Same entry as in 04q250 (Kousseff, 1974).

11q140   Positive band

Jacobs, P. A., Buckton, K. E., Cunningham, C. and
Newton, M. S.: An analysis of the break points
in structural rearrangements in man. J. Med.
Genet. 11:50-64, 1974.
M. R. C. Registry No. K126-60-71 in this report.
46,XY,t(11;19)(q14;q13).

11q141   Positive band

Same entry as in 11p120 (Sanchez, Yunis and
Escobar, 1974).

11q200

Dutrillaux, B.: Chromosomal aspects of human

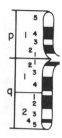

male sterility.   Nobel Symposium 23:205-208, 1972.
46,XY,t(11;22)(q2;q1).

Same entry as in 05p100 (Kadotani et al., 1970).

Same entry as in 05p100 (Singh, Osborne and Wiscovitch, 1973).

11q210   Negative band

Faust, J., Vogel, W. and Loning, B.: A case with 46,XX,del(11)(q21). Clin. Genet. 6:90-97, 1974. Patient H.S. (C 3061) in this report.
46,XX,del(11)(q21).
46,XX,del(11)(pter to q21:).

Same entry as in 01q430 (Jacobs et al., 1974).

Same entry as in 08p120 (Ladda et al., 1974).

11q230   Negative band

Same entry as in 04q350 (de la Chapelle and Schroder, 1973).

Jacobsen, P., Hauge, M., Henningsen, K., Hobloth, N., Mikkelsen, M. and Philip, J.: An (11;21) translocation in four generations with chromosome 11 abnormalities in the offspring. A clinical, cytogenetical, and gene marker study.   Hum. Hered. 23:568-585, 1973.
46,XX and XY,t(11;21)(q23;q22).
46,XX and XY,der(11)der(21)t(11;21)(q23;q22)mat and pat.
Case No. 1 in this report.
46,XX,-11,+der(11)t(11;21)(q23;q22)pat.
Case No. 3 in this report.
46,XY,-21,+der(21)t(11;21)(q23;q22)mat.
46,XY,-21,+der(21)t(11;21)(21pter to 21q22::11q23 to 11qter)mat.

Same entry as in 04q350 (Ockey and de la Chapelle, 1967).

Same entry as in 11p120 (Sanchez, Yunis and Escobar, 1974).

11q240   Positive band

Same entry as in 10q230 (Ferguson-Smith and Page, 1973).

Same entry as in 08p120 (Ladda et al., 1974).

11q250   Negative band

Jacobs, P. A., Buckton, K. E., Cunningham, C. and Newton, M. S.: An analysis of the break points of structural rearrangements in man. J. Med. Genet. 11:50-64, 1974.
M. R. C. Registry No. K186-237-71 in this report.
46,XY,t(11;12)(q25;q13).

Same entry as in 07q110 (Jacobs et al., 1974).

120000

Same entry as in 090000 (Battaglia et al., 1971).

Machin, G. A. and Crolla, J. A.: Chromosome constitution of 500 infants dying during the perinatal period. Humangenetik 23:183-198, 1974. Case No. 24 in this report.
46,XX,t(12q17q).

12p100

Mayeda, K., Weiss, L., Lindahl, R. and Dulby, M.: Localization of the human lactate dehydrogenase B gene on the short arm of chromosome 12. Amer. J. Hum. Genet. 26:59-64, 1974.
46,XX,del(12)(p1).
46,XX,del(12)(qter to p1:).

Same entry as in 01q000 (van den Berghe et al., 1973).

12p110   Negative band

Same entry as in 05p150 (Dewald, Spurbeck and

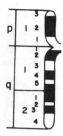

Gordon, 1974).

Friedrich, U. and Nielsen, J.: Autosomal deletions 46,XY,del(12)(p11) and 46,XY/46,XY
del(5)(p13) with no effect on physical or mental
development. Humangenetik 21:127-132, 1974.
Proband No. 9612 in this report.
46,XY,del(12)(p11).
46,XY,del(12)(qter to p11:).

Same entry as in 06q200 (Fryns et al., 1974).

Same entry as in 11p120 (Sanchez, Yunis and
Escobar, 1974).

Same entry as in 08p230 (Uchida and Lin, 1973).

12p130   Negative band

Hamerton, J. L., Ray, M. and Douglas, G. R.:
Chromosome banding techniques in clinical cytogenetics. Nobel Symposium 23:209-213, 1973.
Case IV: TH 140671 WCH-5303 in this report.
46,XX,r(12)(p13q24).
46,XX,r(12)(p13 to q24).

Shapiro, L. R., Graves, Z. R., Warburton, D. and
Huss, H. A.: Autosomal aberrations and gonadal
dysgenesis. Amer. J. Hum. Genet. 26:79A, 1974.
46,XX,tdic(12;14)(p13;p13).
46,XX,tdic(12;14)(12qter to 12p13::14p13 to
14qter).

Warburton, D., Henderson, A. S., Shapiro, L. R.
and Hsu, L. Y. F.: A stable human dicentric
chromosome, tdic(12;14)(p13;p13) including an
intercalary satellite region between centromeres.
Amer. J. Hum. Genet. 25:439-445, 1973.
45,XX,tdic(12;14)(p13;p13).
45,XX,tdic(12;14)(12qter to 12p13::14p13 to
14qter).

12q000

Same entry as in 08q000 (Chen and Woolley, 1971).

Same entry as in 06q200 (Francke, 1972).

Same entry as in 03q100 (Herrmann et al., 1974).

Same entry as in 05p100 (Opitz and Patau, 1974).

Same entry as in 10q000 (Sarto, 1974).

Same entry as in 0Xq000 (Sarto, 1974).

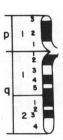

12q100

Same entry as in 09p000 (Guanti et al., 1971).

Same entry as in 02q300 (Shapiro and Warburton, 1972).

12q120   Positive band

Same entry as in 04q260 (Hirschhorn, Lucas and Wallace, 1973).

12q130   Negative band

Same entry as in 11q250 (Jacobs et al., 1974).

12q140   Positive band

Mikkelsen, M.: Rare translocation 47,XY,t(12;21) in Down's syndrome.   Hum. Hered. 24:160-166, 1974.
46,XX and XY,t(12;21)(q14;q22).
47,XY,-12,+der(12)+der(21)t(12;21)[q14;q22)mat.

12q200

Same entry as in 03q100 (Baheux-Morlier, Taillemite and Roux, 1973).

Same entry as in 0Xq200 (Sarto, Therman and Patau, 1973).

12q210   Positive band

Same entry as in 0X0000 (Hamerton et al., 1974).

Same entry as in 01p210 (Sutherland, Bauld and Bain, 1974).

12q240   Negative band

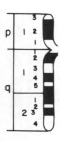

Same entry as in 07q220 (Carpentier, Rethore and Lejeune, 1972).

Faed, M. and Robertson, J.: Integrity of the telomere. Lancet 2:973-974, 1972.
46,XX,t(12;13)(q24;q1).
46,XX,t(12;13)(12pter to 12qter?::13q1 to 13qter;13pter to 13q1::?).
46,XX,-13,+der(13)t(12;13)(q24;q1)mat.
46,XX,-13,+der(13)t(13pter to 13q1::?)mat.

Same entry as in 12p130 (Hamerton, Ray and Douglas, 1973).

Same entry as in 06q100 (Jacobs et al., 1974).

Machin, G. A.: Chromosome abnormality and perinatal death. Lancet 1:549-551, 1974.
46,XX,t(12;17)(q24;q21).

12q241   Negative band

Same entry as in 11p120 (Sanchez, Yunis and Escobar, 1974).

130000

Avirachan, S. and Kajii, T.: Double heteroploidy, 46,XY,t(13q14q),+18, in a spontaneous abortus. Clin. Genet. 4:101-104, 1973.
46,XY,-13,-14,+t(13q14q)+18.

Bhasin, M. K., Foerster, W. and Fuhrmann, W.: A cytogenetic study of recurrent abortion. Humangenetik 18:139-148, 1973.
Case 1 (J. No. 301-71) in this report.
45,XX,t(13q15q).

Borgaonkar, D. S.: Unpublished observations, 1974.
45,XX,t(13q15q).
Subject No. 1633 in this laboratory.
45,XY,der(13q15q)mat.

Borgaonkar, D. S.: Unpublished observations, 1974.
45,XX,t(13q14q).
Subject No. 1901 in this laboratory.

45,XY,der t(13q14q)mat.

Boue, J. and Boue, A.: L'interet en diagnostic prenatal des techniques nouvelles d'identification chromosomique dans des translocations et une aneusomie de recombinaison. Nouv. Presse Med. 2:3097-3102, 1973.
Observation No. 2754 in this report.
46,XX,t(13q15q).

Same entry as in 040000 (Carrel, Sparkes and Wright, 1973).

Caspersson, T., Hulten, M., Lindsten, J., Therkelsen, A. J. and Zech, L.: Identification of different Robertsonian translocations in man by quinacrine mustard fluorescence analysis.
Hereditas 67:213-220, 1971.
Case 3 in this report.
45,XY,t(13q21q).
Cases 5 and 7 in this report.
45,XY,t(13q14q).

Chandley, A. C., Christie, S., Fletcher, J. M., Frackiewicz, A. and Jacobs, P. A.: Translocation heterozygosity and associated subfertility in man. Cytogenetics 11:516-533, 1972.
Patient J. F. (M. R. C. Registry No. K56-183-69) in this report.
45,XY,t(13q14q).
Oligospermia was reported in this patient.

Chandley, A. C. and Fletcher, J. M.: Centromere staining at meiosis in man. Humangenetik 18:247-252, 1973.
M. R. C. Registry No. K19-99-65 in this report.
45,XY,t(13q14q).

Chrz, R., Kozak, J. and Malkova, J.: Densitometric study of G bands of human metaphase chromosomes. Humangenetik 18:149-154, 1973.
t(13q14q).

Dutrillaux, B.: Chromosomal aspects of human male sterility. Nobel Symposium 23:205-208, 1972.
45,XY,t(13q14q).

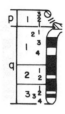

Emberger, J. M., Negre, C. and Lafon, R.: Mosaic trisomy 13 with an isochromosome: 46,XX/46,XX,13-,13qi. Ann. Genet. 15:111-114, 1972.
46,XX/46,XX,-13,i(13q).

Fraccaro, M., Maraschio, P., Pasquali, F., Tiepolo, L., Zuffardi, O. and Giarola, A.: Male infertility and 13/14 translocation. Lancet 1:488, 1973.
45,XY,t(13q14q).

Hecht, F. and Kimberling, W. J.: Patterns of D chromosome involvement in human (DqDq) and (DqGq) Robertsonian rearrangements. Amer. J. Hum. Genet. 23:361-367, 1971.

Jacobs, P. A., Buckton, K. E., Cunningham, C. and Newton, M. S.: An analysis of the break points of structural rearrangements in man. J. Med. Genet. 11:50-64, 1974.
M. R. C. Registry No. K70-212-68 in this report.
46,XX,-13,+t(13q21q).
M. R. C. Registry Nos. K7-80-62, K29-167-66, K46-105-68, K52-226-68, K56-42-69, K93-277-69, K132-270-70, K183-109-71, K204-151-72, K206-158-72 in this report.
45,XX,t(13q14q).
M. R. C. Registry Nos. K-13-86-64, K16-99-65, K18-121-65, K49-162-65, K67-209-66, K32-13-67, K37-205-67, K41-243-67, K44-7-68, K123-131-68, K75-58-70, K139-247-70, K196-47-72 in this report.
45,XY,t(13q14q).
M. R. C. Registry No. K185-229-71 in this report.
45,XX,t(13q22q).
M. R. C. Registry No. K190-281-71 in this report.
45,XY,t(13q22g).

Same entry as in OY0000 (Jones, 1974).

Kistenmacher, M. L., DiGeorge, A. M. and Punnett, H. H.: The association of autoimmune disorders with 18p- syndrome. Amer. J. Hum. Genet. 26:49A, 1974.
45,XX,-13,-18,+t(18q13q).

Newton, M. S., Cunningham, C., Jacobs, P. A., Price, W. H. and Fraser, I. A.: Chromosome

survey of a hospital for the mentally subnormal. Part 2: Autosome abnormalities. Clin. Genet. 3:226-248, 1972.
M. R. C. Registry No. K67-209-66 in this report.
46,XY,-13,-14,+t(13q14q),+21.

Nielsen, J., Hreidarsson, A. B. and Christensen, K. R.: D-D translocations in patients with mental illness. Hereditas 75:131-135, 1973.
45,XX and XY,t(13q14q).

Palmer, C. G., Conneally, P. M. and Christian, J. C.: Translocations of D chromosomes in two families t(13q14q) and t(13q14q)-t(13p14p). J. Med. Genet. 6:166-173, 1969.
Family 1156 in this report.
45,XY,t(13q14q)/46,XY,t(13q14q)t(13p14p).
46,XY,t(13q14q)t(13p14p).

Palmer, C. G., Morris, J. L., Thompson, B. H. and Nance, W. E.: Fertility and 13/14 translocation. Lancet 1:728, 1973.
45,XX and XY,t(13q14q).

Parrington, J. M. and Edwards, J. H.: Patau's syndrome with D1 duplication-deficiency derived from a maternal D group pericentric inversion. Ann. Hum. Genet. 35:35-45, 1971.

Parslow, M. I., Gardner, R. J. M. and Veale, A. M. O.: Giemsa banding in the t(13q14q) carrier mother of a translocation trisomy 13 abortus. Humangenetik 18:183-184, 1973.
45,XX,t(13q13q).
46,XX,-13,+der t(13q13q)mat.

Raaijmakers-Engeln, E.: Identification of D/D translocations in mentally retarded patients. Humangenetik 17:165-168, 1973.
45,XX,t(13q14q).
45,XY,t(13q15q).

Scheres, J. M. J. C.: Identification of two Robertsonian translocations with a Giemsa banding technique. Humangenetik 15:253-256, 1972.
Case 1 in this report.
46,XY,-13,-14,+t(13q14q),+21.

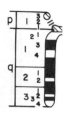

Singh, D. N., Osborne, R. A. and Horger, E. O.: A case of double aneuploidy of Down's syndrome and familial 13q and 14q translocation. Amer. J. Hum. Genet. 26:81A, 1974.
45,XX,t(13q14q).
46,XY,-13,-14,+der t(13q14q)mat,+21.

Stoll, C. and Levy, J. M.: Identification of a familial Robertsonian translocation t(13q14q) by means of thermic moderated denaturation. Humangenetik 19:211-214, 1973.
45,XX,t(13q14q).

Wennstrom, J. and Schroder, J.: A t(13q14q) family with the translocation and a Philadelphia chromosome in one member. Humangenetik 20:71-73, 1973.
45,XX,t(13q14q),del(22)(q1:).
45,XX and XY,der t(13q14q)mat and pat.

Wilson, J. A.: Fertility in balanced heterozygotes for a familial centric fusion translocation, t(DqDq). J. Med. Genet. 8:175-178, 1971.
45,XX,t(13q14q).

Zeuthen, E. and Nielsen, J.: D-D translocations in males examined for military service. J. Med. Genet. 10:356-361, 1973.
Propositus Nos. 4060 and 5043 in this report.
45,XY,t(13q14q).

13p100   Variable band

Coffin, G. S. and Wilson, M. G.: Ring chromosome D(13). Amer. J. Dis. Child. 119:370-373, 1970.
46,XX,r(13).

Fitzgerald, P. H.: Ring chromosome 13 and haptoglobin heterozygosity. Clin. Genet. 4:25-27, 1973.
46,XX and XY,r(13).
Evidence is presented against any claim that the Hp locus is situated on the long arm of chromosome 13.

Same entry as in 01p000 (Francke, 1972).

Fryns, J. P., Deroover, J., Cassiman, J. J.,

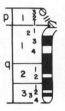

Goffaux, P., Lebas, E. and van den Berghe, H.:
Malformative syndrome with ring chromosome 13.
Humangenetik 24:235-240. 1974.
Case GF 090953 in this report.
46,XY,r(13).

Same entry as in 08q210 (Fryns et al., 1974).

Grace, E., Drennan, J., Colver, D. and Gordon, R.
R.: The 13q- deletion syndrome. J. Med. Genet.
8:351-357, 1971.
46,XX and XY,r(13).

Hauksdottir, H., Halldorsson, S., Jensson, O.,
Mikkelsen, M. and McDermott, A.: Pericentric
inversion of chromosome 13 in a large family
leading to duplication deficiency causing congenital malformations in three individuals. J.
Med. Genet. 9:413-421, 1972.
46,XX and XY,inv(13)(p1q2).
46,XX and XY,inv(13)(pter to p1::q2 to p1::q2 to
qter).

Hollowell, J. G., Littlefield, L. G., Dharmkrong-
At, A., Folger, G. M., Heath, C. F. and Bloom, G.
E.: Ring 13 chromosome with normal haptoglobin
inheritance. J. Med. Genet. 8:222-226, 1971.
46,XX,r(13).
Chromosome identification by autoradiography.

Kistenmacher, M. L. and Punnett, H. H.: Comparative behavior of ring chromosomes. Amer. J. Hum.
Genet. 22:304-318, 1969.
Case II (G.C. SCHC No. 6404006) in this report.
46,XX,r(13).

Lindenbaum, R. H., Blackwell, N. L. and de Sa, D.
J.: A case of double aneuploidy, 47,XXY,14-
,t(13q14q)+, also probably homozygous for the
cystic fibrosis gene. J. Med. Genet. 9:232-235,
1972.
47,XXY,-14,+t(13;14)(p1;q1).
47,XXY,-14,+t(13;14)(13qter to 13p1::14q1 to
14qter).

Mellman, W. J.: Personal Communication, 1974.
46,XX,r(13).
Mutant Cell Repository No. GM-250.

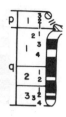

Mikelsaar, A. V. N., Tuur, S. J. and Kyaosaar, M. E.: Human karyotype polymorphism. I. Routine and fluorescence microscopic investigation of chromosomes in a normal adult population. Humangenetik 20:89-101, 1973.

Same entry as in 05p100 (Niebuhr, 1972).

Niebuhr, E.: Unusual findings by fluorescence microscopy at a t(13q14q). Humangenetik 15:96-98, 1972.
46,XX and XY,tdic(13;14)(p1;p1).
The author suggests that Robertsonian translocations in man could be due to breaks in the short arms of the involved chromosomes.

Niebuhr, E. and Ottosen, J.: Ring chromosome D(13) associated with multiple congenital malformations. Ann. Genet. 16:157-166, 1973.

Nielsen, J., Friedrich, U. and Hreidarsson, A. B.: Frequency of deletion of short arm satellites on acrocentric chromosomes. J. Med. Genet. 11:177-180, 1974.
Father of propositus No. 6450 in this report.
46,XY,13ps-.
Propositus No. 6450 in this report.
46,XX,der(13ps-)pat.
Mother of propositus No. 8928 in this report.
46,XX,13ps-.
Propositus 8928 in this report.
46,XY,der(13ps-)mat.
Propositus No. 12579 in this report.
46,XY,13ps-).
Mother and maternal uncle of propositus No. 12850 in this report.
46,XX and XY,13ps-.
Propositus No. 12850 in this report.
46,XY,der(13ps-)mat.

Nielsen, J., Friedrich, U., Hreidarsson, A. B., Noel, B., Quack, B. and Mottet, J.: Brilliantly fluorescing enlarged short arms D or G. Lancet 1:1049-1050, 1974.

Salamanca, F., Buentello, L. and Armendares, S.: Ring D1 chromosome with remarkable morphological variation in a boy with mental retardation. Ann.

Genet. 15:183-186, 1972.
46,XY,r(13).

Same entry as in 07p000 (Wilson et al., 1973).

Zink, U., Rix, R., Grosse, K. P. and Schwanitz,
G.: Ring chromosom D13. Kasuistik und Uber-
sicht. Klin. Paediat. 185:192-197, 1973.
46,XX,r(13).

13p110   Variable band

Cantu, J. M., Salamanca, F., Sanchez, J., Pena,
T., Pacheco, C. and Armendares, S.: Human
acrocentric rings and "satellite" association.
Amer. J. Hum. Genet. 26:18A, 1974.
Case C in this report.
46,XY,r(13)(p11q?).

Same entry as in 01q110 (Hirschhorn, Lucas and
Wallace, 1973).

Kreiger, D., Palmer, C. and Biegel, A.: Human
autosomal deletion mapping and HL-A. Humangenetik 23:159-160, 1974.
45,XX,-13,-14,+t(13;14)(p11;p11).
46,XX,t(13;14)(p11;p11).
46,XX,r(13)(p11q14).

Same entry as in 05q110 (Leisti, 1974).

Same entry as in 01q110 (Lucas and Wallace,
1972).

13p120   Variable band

Hsu, L. Y. F., Kim, H. J., Sujansky, E., Kousseff, B. and Hirschhorn, K.: Reciprocal translocation versus centric fusion between two No. 13
chromosomes. A case of 46,XX,-13,+
t(13;13)(p12;q13) and a case of 46,XY,-13,+
t(13;13)(p12;p12). Cytogenet. Cell Genet.
12:235-244, 1973.
Case a in this report.
46,XX,-13,+t(13;13)(p12;q13).
Case b in this report.
46,XY,-13,+t(13;13)(p12;p12).

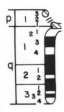

Niebuhr, E.:   Dicentric and monocentric Robert-sonian translocations in man.   Humangenetik 16:217-226, 1972.
Case 1 in this report.
45,XX,tdic(13;13) (p12:p12).
45,XX,tdic(13;13) (13qter to 13p12::13p12 to 13qter).
Case 2 in this report.
45,XX,tdic(13;14) (p12;p11 or 12).
45,XX,tdic(13;14) (13qter to 13p12::14p11 or 14p12 to 14qter).

Niebuhr, E.:   Reexamination of a family with a + (13q14q) and a ring D(13) child. Ann. Genet. 16:199-202, 1973.
46,XY,r(13) (p12q33).
46,XY,r(13) (p12 to q33).

Taysi, K., Bobrow, M., Balci, S., Madan, K., Metin, A. and Burhan, S.: Duplication/deficiency product of a pericentric inversion in man. A cause of D1 trisomy syndrome. J. Pediat. 82:263-268, 1973.
46,XX,inv(13) (p12q14).
46,XX,inv(13) (pter to p12::q14 to p12::q14 to qter).

13q000

Allderdice, P. W., Davis, J. G., Miller, O. J., Klinger, H. P., Warburton, D., Miller, D. A., Allen, F. H., Abrams, C. A. L. and McGilvray, E.: The 13q- deletion syndrome.   Amer. J. Hum. Genet. 21:499-512, 1969.

Bochkov, N. P., Kuleshov, N. P., Chebotarev, A. N., Alekhin, V. I. and Midian, S. A.: Population cytogenetic investigation of newborns in Moscow. Humangenetik 22:139-152, 1974.
46,XX,del(13q-).

Same entry as in 05p100 (Carpentier et al., 1972).

Carrel, R. E., Sparkes, R. S. and Wright, S. W.: Partial F trisomy associated with familial F/13 translocation detected and identified by parental chromosome studies. J. Pediat. 78:664-672, 1971.

46,XY,t(13q-;Fp+).
46,XX,der(13)der(F)t(13q-;Fp+)pat.
46,XX and XY,-13,+der(13)t(13q-;Fp+)mat.
Patients L.C.R., P.L.R. and W.E.R. in this
report.
46,XX and XY,-13,+der(13)t(13;F)(13pter to
13q::Fp to Fpter)mat.

Same entry as in 05q000 (Fredga and Hall, 1970).

Same entry as in 06q200 (Fryns et al., 1974).

Same entry as in 02q000 (Genest et al., 1971).

Same entry as in 0Yq100 (Gilgenkrantz, Pierson
and Mauuary, 1973).

Grosse, K. P. and Schwanitz, G.: A new syndrome
caused by deletion of a part of a chromosome
(13q-). Case descriptions and compilation of
symptoms. Klin. Paediat. 185:468-473, 1973.
46,XY,del(13)(q).
46,XY,del(13)(pter to q:).

Hayes, T. G. and del Rosario, A. J.: D-group
chromosomal aberration: 13q+. Lancet 2:1215,
1973.
46,XX,13q+.

Martin, P. A., Thorburn, M. J. and Smith-Read, E.
H. M.: Chromosomal rearrangements in three
generations of a Jamaican family. Cytogenetics
9:360-368, 1970.
46,XX,ins(17;13)(q;q).
46,XX,ins(17;13)(17qter to 17q::13q to 13q::17q
to 17pter;13pter to 13q::13q to 13qter).
46,XX and XY,der(17)der(13)ins(17;13)(q;q)mat.

McGilvray, E., Kajii, T., Freund, M., Bamatter,
F. and Klein, D.: A balanced 13-18 translocation
[46,XY,t(13q-;18q+)] in the father of an infant
with multiple anomalies. Humangenetik 12:316-
322, 1971.
46,XY,t(13;18)(q;q2).
Chromosome identification by autoradiography.

Neu, R. L. and Gardner, L. I.: Three families
with abnormal inherited chromosomes: 2q+mat,t(Cp+

; 13q-) mat   and t (3?-; 5q+) pat.   Ann. Genet. 15: 19-
23, 1971.
46,XX,t(Cp+;13q-).
Case No. 2 in this report.
46,XX,der(C)der(13)t(Cp+;13q-)mat.

Same entry as in 01p000 (Newton et al., 1972).

O'Grady, R. B., Rothstein, T. B. and Romano, P.
E.:   D-group deletion syndromes and retinoblastoma. Amer. J. Ophthal. 77:40-45, 1974.
46,XX,Dq-.
Although no specific identification has been made
of the chromosome and the segment deleted, it is
assumed that the chromosome is 13 and a terminal
deletion of about half of the long arm is present.

Same entry as in 09q000 (Rary et al., 1974).

Same entry as in 04p100 (Taillemite et al.,
1973).

Talvik, T. A., Mikelsaar, A. V. N., Mikelsaar,
R., Kyaosaar, M. E. and Tuur, S. J.: Inherited
translocations in two families (t(14q+;10q-) and
t(13q-;21q+)). Humangenetik 19:215-226, 1973.
Family F2 in this report.
46,XX and XY,t(13;21)(q;q2).
46,XX,t(21q+).
46,XY,-21,+der t(13;21)(q;q2)pat.
46,XY,-21,+der t(13;21)(21pter to 21q2::13q to
13qter)pat.

Wilson, M. G., Towner, J. W. and Fujimoto, A.:
Retinoblastoma and D-chromosome deletions. Amer.
J. Hum. Genet. 25:57-61, 1973.

13q100

Same entry as in 12q240 (Faed and Robertson,
1972).

Pasquali, F., Zuffardi, O., Severi, F., Colombo,
A. and Burgio, G. R.: Tandem translocation 15/
13. Ann. Genet. 16:47-50, 1973.
45,XY,tan(13;15)(q1;q2).
45,XY,-13,tan(13;15)(15pter to 15q2::13q1 to

13qter).

13q120   Negative band

Same entry as in 0Xq270 (Crandall et al., 1974).

Same entry as in 09q220 (Howard, Yarbrough and Stoddard, 1974).

Same entry as in 06p110 (Jacobs et al., 1974).

von Koskull, H. and Aula, P.: Inherited (13;14) translocation and reproduction. Report on three families. Humangenetik 24:85-91, 1974.
Family A in this report.
46,XY,t(13;14)(q12;q12).
46,XY,t(13;14)(13pter to 13q12::14q12 to 14qter;14pter to 14q12::13q12 to 13qter).
46,XX,der(13)der(14)t(13;14)(q12;q12) pat.
46,XX,-14,+der(14)t(13;14)(q12;q12) mat.
46,XX,-14,+der(14)t(13;14)(14pter to 14q12::13q12 to 13qter) mat.
Family B in this report.
46,XX,t(13;14)(q12;q12).
46,XX,t(13;14)(13pter to 13q12::14q12 to 14qter;14pter to 14q12::13q12 to 13qter).
Family C in this report.
46,XX and XY,t(13;14)(q12;q12).
46,XX and XY,t(13;14)(13pter to 13q12::14q12 to 14qter;14pter to 14q12::13q12 to 13qter).
46,XX and XY,der(13)der(14)t(13;14)(q12;q12) mat and pat.
47,XX,der(13)der(14)t(13;14)(q12;q12) pat,+21.

13q130   Positive band

Same entry as 13p120 (Hsu, et al., 1973, Case a).

13q140   Negative band

Same entry as in 04p140 (Jacobs et al., 1974).

Same entry as in 04q310 (Jenkins, Curcuru-Giordano and Krishna, 1974).

Same entry as in 03q290 (Kreiger, Palmer and Biegel, 1974).

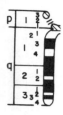

Same entry as in 13p110 (Kreiger, Palmer and Biegel, 1974).

Orye, E., Delbeke, M. J. and Vandenabeele, B.: Retinoblastoma and long arm deletion of chromosome 13. Attempts to define the deleted segment. Clin. Genet. 5:457-464, 1974.
46,XX,del(13)(q14q22).
46,XX,del(13)(pter to q14::q22 to qter).

Same entry as in 09q220 (Rary, 1974).

Schinzel, A., Schmid, W. and Murset, G.: Different forms of incomplete trisomy 13, mosaicism and partial trisomy for the proximal and distal long arm. Report of three cases. Humangenetik 22:287-298, 1974.
Mother of Cases 2 and 3 in this report.
46,XX,t(13;17)(q14;p13).
46,XX,t(13;17)(13pter to 13q14::17p13 to 17pter;17qter to 17p13::13q14 to 13qter).
Case 2 in this report.
46,XY,-17,+der(17)t(13;17)(q14;p13)mat.
Case 3 in this report.
47,XY,+der(13)t(13;17)(q14;p13)mat.

Same entry as in 13p120 (Taysi et al., 1973).

Wilroy, R. S., Summitt, R. L. and Martens, P. R.: Partial trisomy for different segments of chromosome 13 in several individuals of the same family. Newport Beach, Calif., Birth Defects Conf., National Foundation - March of Dimes, p. 89, June 16-21, 1974.
46,XX,t(13;17)(q14;p11).
46,XX,t(13;17)(13pter to 13q14::17p11 to 17pter;17qter to 17p11::13q14 to 13qter).

13q200

Same entry as in 13p100 (Hauksdottir et al., 1972).

13q210   Positive band

Same entry as in 11q130 (Jacobs et al, 1974a and 1974b).

13q220   Negative band

Ikeuchi, T., Sonta, S., Sasaki, M., Hujita, M.
and Tsunematsu, K.: Chromosome banding patterns
in an infant with 13q-   syndrome. Humangenetik
21:309-314, 1974.
46,XY,der(13)del(13)(q22)mat.
46,XY,der(13)del(13)(pter to q12: mat.

Same entry as in 01p130 (Jacobs et al., 1974).

Same entry as in 13q140 (Orye, Delbeke and
Vandenabeele, 1974).

13q300

Francke, U.: Quinacrine mustard fluorescence of
human chromosomes: characterization of unusual
translocations. Amer. J. Hum. Genet. 24:189-213,
1972.
46,XX,t(13;20)(q3;p1).
46,XX and XY,-13,+der(13)t(13;20)(q3;p1)mat.
46,XX and XY,-13,+der(13)t(13;20)(13pter to
13q3::20p1 to 20pter)mat.
Case 11: LR 082262 in this report.
46,XX,-13,+der(13)t(13;20)(q3;p1)mat.
46,XX,-13,+der(13)t(13;20)(13pter to 13q3::20p1
to 20pter)mat.

Same entry as in 08q000 (Khudr et al., 1973).

Same entry as in 11q100 (Rott et al., 1972).

13q310   Positive band

Same entry as in 03q100 (Jacobs et al., 1974).

13q330   Positive band

Same entry as in 02q320 (Forabosco et al., 1973).

Same entry as in 13p120 (Niebuhr, 1973).

13q340   Negative band

Same entry as in 11p120 (Sanchez, Yunis and
Escobar, 1974).

Same entry as in 04q200 (Schrott et al., 1974).

Same entry as in 01q320 (Steffensen, 1974).

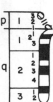 140000

Same entry as in 130000 (Avirachan and Kajii, 1973).

Same entry as in 130000 (Borgaonkar, 1974).

Boue, J. and Boue, A.: L'interet en diagnostic prenatal des techniques nouvelles d'identification chromosomique dans des translocations et une aneusomie de recombinaison. Nouv. Presse Med. 2:3097-3102, 1973.
Observation No. 2400 LA90, and LA92 in this report.
t(14q21q).

Caspersson, T., Hulten, M., Lindsten, J., Therkelsen, A. J. and Zech, L.: Identification of different Robertsonian translocations in man by quinacrine mustard fluorescence analysis. Hereditas 67:213-220, 1971.
Cases 1, 2 and 4 in this report.
45,XY,t(14q21q).
Case 6 in this report.
45,XY,t(14q14q).

Same entry as in 130000 (Caspersson et al., 1971).

Same entry as in 090000 (Centerwall et al., 1974).

Same entry as in 130000 (Chandley et al., 1972).

Chrz, R., Kozak, J. and Malkova, J.: Densitometric study of G bands of human metaphase chromosomes. Humangenetik 18:149-154, 1973.
t(14q21q).

Same entry as in 130000 (Chrz, Kozak and Malkova, 1973).

Same entry as in 130000 (Dutrillaux, 1972).

Dutrillaux, B.:   Chromosomal aspects of human
male sterility.   Nobel Symposium 23:205-208,
1972.
45,XY,t(14q21q).

Same entry as in 130000 (Fraccaro et al., 1973).

Same entry as in 060000 (Jacobs et al., 1974).

Same entry as in 130000 (Jacobs et al., 1974).

Jacobs, P. A., Buckton, K. E., Cunningham, C. and
Newton, M. S.: An analysis of the break points
of structural rearrangements in man. J. Med.
Genet. 11:50-64, 1974.
M. R. C. Registry No. K217-228-72 in this report.
45,XY,t(14q15q).
M. R. C. Registry Nos. K71-197-68, K130-92-68,
K107-10-71 and K159-173-71 in this report.
45,XX,t(14q21q).
M. R. C. Registry No. K61-96-69 in this report.
45,XY,t(14q21q).
M. R. C. Registry Nos. K2-85-61, K169-213-68 and
K165-175-69 in this report.
46,XX,-14,+t(14q21q).
M. R. C. Registry Nos. K1-84-61, K152-86-61, K6-
73-62, K33-52-67, 157-221-70 and K168-279-70 in
this report.
46,XY,-14+t(14q21q).
M. R. C. Registry No. K141-107-71 in this report.
45,XY,t(14q22q).

Lubs, H. A. and Ruddle, F. H.: Chromosomal
abnormalities in the human population: estimation
of rates based on New Haven newborn study.
Science 169:495-497, 1970.
Cytogenet. Cell Genet. 12:368-369, 1973.
45,XX,t(14q22q).
Mutant Cell Repository No. GM-5.

Neu, R. L., Valentine, F. A. and Gardner, L. I.:
Segregation of a t(14q22q) chromosome in a large
kindred. Amer. J. Hum. Genet. 26:63A, 1974.
45,XX and XY,t(14q22q).
A large kindred in which 21 members are balanced
carriers is reported.

Same entry as in 130000 (Newton et al., 1972).

Same entry as in 130000 (Nielsen, Hreidarsson and Christensen, 1973).

Same entry as in 130000 (Palmer, Conneally and Christian, 1969).

Same entry as in 130000 (Palmer et al., 1973).

Same entry as in 130000 (Raaijmakers-Engeln, 1973).

Same entry as in 130000 (Singh, Osborne and Horger, 1974).

Same entry as in 130000 (Stoll and Levy, 1973).

Same entry as in 130000 (Wennstrom and Schroder, 1973).

Same entry as in 130000 (Wilson, 1971).

Zeuthen, E. and Nielsen, J.: D-D translocations in males examined for military service. J. Med. Genet. 10:356-361, 1973.
Propositus No. 2800 in this report.
45,XY,t(14q15q).

Same entry as in 130000 (Zeuthen and Nielsen, 1973).

14p100   Variable band

Bauchinger, M. and Schmid, E.: A case with balanced (14p+;15p-) translocation. Humangenetik 8:312-320, 1970.
46,XY,t(14p+;15p-).
Chromosome identification by autoradiography.

Emerit, I., Noel, B., Thiriet, M., Loubon, M. and Quack, B.: Short arm deletion of chromosome 14. Humangenetik 15:33-38, 1972.
46,XY,del(14)(p1).
46,XY,del(14)(qter to p1:).

Gigliani, F., de Capoa, A. and Rocchi, A.: A marker number 14 with double satellite observed in two generations. Humangenetik 15:191-195, 1972.

46,XY,t(D or G;14)(p1;p1).
46,XX,der(D or G)der(14)t(D or G;14)(p1;p1).

Gilgenkrantz, S., Cabrol, C., Lausecker, C.,
Hartbeyler, M. E. and Bohe, B.: The Dr syndrome.
Report of a new case (46,XX,14r). Ann. Genet.
14:23-31, 1971.
46,XX,r(14).
Chromosome identification by autoradiography.

Same entry as in 05q100 (Knight, Sakaguchi and
Luzzatti, 1971).

Mikelsaar, A. V. N., Tuur, S. J. and Kyaosaar, M.
E.: Human karyotype polymorphism. I. Routine and
fluorescence microscopic investigation of chromosomes in a normal adult population. Humangenetik
20:89-101, 1973.

Same entry as in 13p100 (Niebuhr, 1972).

Same entry as in 13p120 (Niebuhr, 1972, case No.
2).

Nielsen, J., Friedrich, U. and Hreidarsson, A.
B.: Frequency of deletion of short arm satellites in acrocentric chromosomes. J. Med. Genet.
11:177-180, 1974.
46,XY,14ps-.
Propositus No. 10903 in this report.
46,XY,der(14ps-)pat.

Thorburn, M. J. and Martin, P. A.: Chromosome
studies in 101 mentally retarded handicapped
children. J. Med. Genet. 8:59-64, 1971.
46,XX,14p+.
46,XY,der(14p+)mat.

14p110   Variable band

Jacobs, P. A., Buckton, K. E., Cunningham, C. and
Newton, M. S.: An analysis of the break points
in structural rearrangements in man. J. Med.
Genet. 11:50-64, 1974.
M. R. C. Registry No. K20-138-65 in this report.
46,XX,t(14;21)(p11;p1).

Kreiger, D., Palmer, C. and Biegel, A.: Human

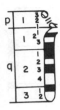

autosomal deletion mapping and HL-A. Humangenetik 23:159-160, 1974.
46,XX,t(14;20)(p11;g11).

Same entry as in 13p110 (Kreiger, Palmer and
Biegel, 1974).

14p120   Variable band

Rocchi, A., de Capoa, A. and Gigliani, F.:
Double satellites: Autoradiographic study of a
chromosomal marker observed in two generations.
Humangenetik 14:6-12, 1971.
46,XX,t(14;15)(p12p13).
46,XX,t(14;15)(14qter to 14p12::?;15qter to
15p13::14p12 to 14pter).
46,XX,der(14)der(15)t(14;15)(p12;p13)mat.

14p130   Variable band

Same entry as in 12p130 (Shapiro et al., 1974).

Same entry as in 12p130 (Warburton et al., 1973).

14q000

Same entry as in 0Xq000 (Allderdice et al.,
1971).

Same entry as in 05p100 (Breg et al., 1972).

Same entry as in 01q000 (Buckton, 1972).

Krompotic, E., Rosenthal, I. M., Szego, K. and
Bocian, M.:   Trisomy F(?20). Report of a 14q-
F(?20) familial translocation.   Ann. Genet.
14:291-299, 1971.
46,XY,t(14q-;?20q+).
47,XY,der(14)der(20)t(14q-;20q+)pat,+20.

Same entry as in 0Yp110 (Krompotic et al., 1972).

Same entry as in 05p100 (Miller et al., 1971).

Same entry as in 03q000 (Neu, Barlow and Gardner,
1973).

Orye, E. and van Nevel, C.:   Familial D/E trans-

location.   Humangenetik 6:191-199, 1968.
46,XX,t(14;17)(q;q2).
46,XX,der(14)der(17)t(14;17)(q;q2)mat.
47,XX,+der(14)t(14;17)(q;q2)mat.

Same entry as in 02q000 (Reisman and Kasahara, 1968).

Same entry as in 02q000 (Reiss et al., 1972).

Same entry as in 010000 (Surana et al., 1974).

Talvik, T. A., Mikelsaar, A. V. N. and Mikelsaar, R. V. A.: Familial translocation between chromosomes of groups C and D [46,t(Cq-;Dq+)]. Genetika 8:123-132, 1972.
46,XX,t(Cq-;14q+).
46,XX and XY,der(C)der(14)t(Cq-;14q+)mat and pat.
Patient V. I. in this report.
46,XY,14q+.
"The patient was an infant boy with mental retardation and growth defects who was partially trisomic for the long arm of chromosome C10 (or C11) and partially monosomic for the distal part of the long arm of chromosome 14."

14q100

Fryns, J. P., Cassiman, J. J. and van den Berghe, H.:   Tertiary partial 14 trisomy 47,XX,+14q-. Humangenetik 24:71-77, 1974
46,XX,t(14;19)(q1;19+).
Diana W. 141065 in this report.
47,XX,+der(14)t(14q-;19+).
Further identification for chromosome 19 region in this report is lacking.

Same entry as in 13p100 (Lindenbaum, Blackwell and de Sa, 1972).

14q110   Negative band

Same entry as in 09q340 (Danilowicz, Feingold and Wolman, 1973).

14q120   Positive band

Same   entry as in 07p130 (Cooledge, Beatty-DeSana

and Hoggard, 1974).

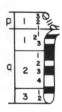

Hecht, F., McCaw, B. K. and Koler, R. D.:
Ataxia-telangiectasia-clonal growth of translocation lymphocytes. New Eng. J. Med. 289:286-291,
1973.
46,XY,t(14;14)(q12;q31).

Laurent, C., Dutrillaux, B., Biemont, M. A.,
Genoud, J. and Bethenod, M.: Translocation
t(14q-;21q+) chez le pere. Trisomie 14 et monosomie 21 partielles chez la fille. Ann. Genet.
16:281-284, 1973.
46,XY,t(14;21)(q12;q22).
46,XY,t(14;21)(14pter to 14q12::21q22 to
21qter;21pter to 21q22::14q12 to 14qter).
46,XX,-21,+der(21)t(14;21)(q12;q22)pat.
46,XX,-21,+der(21)t(14;21)(21pter to 21q22::14q12
to 14qter)pat.

Same entry as in 13q120 (von Koskull and Aula,
1974).

14q130   Negative band

Same entry as in 07p130 (Cooledge, Beatty-DeSana
and Hoggard, 1974).

14q200

Same entry as in 06q210 (Allderdice et al.,
1971).

Same entry as in 07q300 (de la Chapelle, Schroder
and Kokkonen, 1973).

Same entry as in 0Yp110 (Krompotic et al., 1972).

Muldal, S., Enoch, B. A., Ahmed, A. and Harris,
R.: Partial trisomy 14q- and pseudoxanthoma
elasticum. Clin. Genet. 4:480-489, 1973.
47,XX,+14q-.
47,XX,+?del(14)(q2).

Pfeiffer, R. A., Buttinghaus, K. and Struck, H.:
Partial trisomy 14 following a balanced reciprocal translocation t(14q-;21q+). Humangenetik
20:187-189, 1973.

46,XY,t(14;21)(q22 or q23;q22).
46,XY,t(14;21)(14pter to 14q22 or 23::21q22 to
21qter;21pter to 21q22::14q22 or 23 to 14qter).
46,XX,-21,+der(21)t(14;21)(q22 or q23;q22)pat.
46,XX,-21,+der(21)t(14;21)(21pter to 21q22::14q22
or 23 to 14qter)pat.

Same entry as in 09p200 (Short, Solitaire and
Breg, 1972).

14q210   Positive band

Same entry as in 05p140 (Borgaonkar et al.,
1973).

14q220   Negative band

Fawcett, W. A., McCord, W. K. and Francke, U.:
Trisomy 14q-. Newport Beach, Calif., Birth
Defects Conf., National Foundation - March of
Dimes, p. 90, June 16-21, 1974.
46,XX,t(14;20)(q22;q13).
46,XX,t(14;20)(14pter to 14q22::20q13 to
20qter;20pter to 20q13::14q22 to 14qter).
47,XX,+der t(14;20)(q22;q13)mat.
47,XX,+der t(14;20)(14pter to 14q22::20q13 to
20qter)mat.

14q230   Positive band

Same entry as in 01q420 (Jacobs et al., 1974).

14q300

Same entry as in 0Xp110 (Buckton et al., 1971).

Same entry as in 11q100 (Nakagome, Iinuma and
Matsui, 1973).

Same entry as in 10q200 (Talvik et al., 1973).

14q310   Negative band

Same entry as in 14q120 (Hecht, McCaw and Koler,
1973).

14q320   Negative band

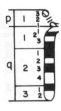

Same entry as in 07q310 (Alfi, Donnell and Kramer, 1973).

Same entry as in 0Xp110 (Buckton et al., 1971).

Same entry as in 0Xp110 (Jacobs et al., 1974).

Same entry as in 07q110 (Lozzio and Klepper, 1974).

Same entry as in 0Xq130 (Opitz, Pallister and Ruddle, 1973).

150000

Same entry as in 090000 (Baccichetti and Tenconi, 1973).

Same entry as in 130000 (Bhasin, Foerster and Fuhrmann, 1973).

Same entry as in 130000 (Borgaonkar, 1974).

Same entry as in 130000 (Boue and Boue, 1973).

Same entry as in 0Yq100 (Friedrich and Nielsen, 1972).

Friedrich, U., Nielsen, J. and Sehested, J.: A family with 15-22 translocation. Hereditas 72:172-174, 1972.
45,XX,t(15q22q).
45,XX and XY,der t(15q22q)mat.

Jackson, L. and Barr, M.: A 45,XY,5-,15-, t(5q15q) cri du chat child. J. Med. Genet. 7:161-163, 1970.
45,XY,t(5q15q).

Same entry as in 140000 (Jacobs et al., 1974).

Jacobs, P. A., Buckton, K. E., Cunningham, C. and Newton, M. S.: An analysis of the break points of structural rearrangements in man. J. Med. Genet. 11:50-64, 1974.
M. R. C. Registry No. K22-1-66 in this report.
46,XX,-15,+t(15q21q).
M. R. C. Registry Nos. K38-204-67 and K142-384-67

in this report.
45,XY,t(15q22q).

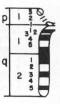

Same entry as in 100000 (Lewandovsky, Sanchez and
Yunis, 1974).

Lucas, M.: Translocation between both members of
chromosome pair number 15 causing recurrent
abortions. Ann. Hum. Genet. 32:347-352, 1969.
45,XX,t(15q15q).
46,XY,-15,+der(15)t(15q15q)mat.
Chromosome identification by autoradiography.

Podugolnikova, O. A. and Batienko, G. S.:
Cytogenetic study of a family with an aberrant
inv(15p+q-) chromosome inherited through five
generations. Genetika 8:129-137, 1972.
46,XX,inv(15)(pq).
46,XX and XY,inv(15)(pq)mat.
46,XX,inv(15)(pq)mat,inv(15)(pq)?pat.
Patient S. A. in this report.
46,XY,inv(15)(pq)mat.

Same entry as in 130000 (Raaijmakers-Engeln,
1973).

Same entry as in 140000 (Zeuthen and Nielsen,
1973).

15p100   Variable band

Bannerman, R. M., Marinello, M. J., Cohen, M. M.
and Lockwood, C.:   A family with an inherited
marker chromosome (46,D-,mar15-). Amer. J. Hum.
Genet. 23:281-188, 1971.

Same entry as in 14p100 (Bauchinger and Schmid,
1970).

Crandall, B. F., Carrel, R. E. and Sparkes, R.
S.: Chromosome findings in 700 children referred
to a psychiatric clinic. J. Pediat. 80:62-68,
1972.
Patient D. R. in this report.
46,XY,inv(15)(pq).

Crandall, B. F. and Sparkes, R. S.: Pericentric inversion of a number 15 chromosome in nine members of one family. Cytogenetics 9:307-316, 1970.
46,XX and XY,inv(15)(pq).
46,XX and XY,der(15)inv(15)(pq)mat and pat.

Emberger, J. M., Rossi, D., Jean, R., Bounet, H. and Dumas, R.: A ring D chromosome (46,XY,15r). Humangenetik 11:295-299, 1971.
46,XY,r(15).
The ring chromosome was identified as No. 15 by autoradiography.

Forabosco, A., Dutrillaux, B., Vazzoler, G. and Lejeune, J.: Ring chromosome 15: r(15) identification by controlled heating. Ann. Genet. 15:267-270, 1972.
46,XY,r(15).

Same entry as in 10q200 (Francke, 1972).

Same entry as in 0Yq100 (Friedrich and Nielsen, 1972).

Same entry as in 0Yq100 (Frund et al., 1972).

German, J.: Studying chromosomes today. Amer. Sci. 58:182-201, 1970.
46,XY,15p+.
46,XY,der(15p+)pat.

Hahnemann, N. and Eiberg, H.: Antenatal genetic diagnosis in a kindred with a 15p+ chromosome. Clin. Genet. 4:464-473, 1973.
"The marker chromosome could represent a Y/15 translocation, as judged from morphology and an intensive fluorescence of extra materials or it could possibly be interpreted as a giant satellite."

Machin, G. A.: Chromosome abnormality and perinatal death. Lancet 1:549-551, 1974.
46,XX,15p+.

Machin, G. A. and Crolla, J. A.: Chromosome constitution of 500 infants dying during the perinatal period. Humangenetik 23:183-198, 1974.

Case No. 27 in this report.
46,XX,15p+.

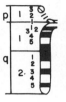

Mikelsaar, A. V. N., Tuur, S. J. and Kyaosaar, M. E.: Human karyotype polymorphism. I. Routine and fluorescence microscopic investigation of chromosomes in a normal adult population. Humangenetik 20:89-101, 1973.

Nielsen, J., Friedrich, U., Hreidarsson, A. B., Noel, B., Quack, B. and Mottet, J.: Brilliantly fluorescing enlarged short arms D or G. Lancet 1:1049-1050, 1974.

Same entry as in 0Yq110 (Pfeiffer et al., 1973).

Stoll, C., Paira, M. and Levy, J. M.: 15p+ familial chromosome with multiple malformations in a new-born child. Ann. Pediat. 21:179-183, 1974.
46,XY,15p+.
The familial 15p+ chromosome was present in clinically normal relatives.

Therkelsen, A. J., Petersen, G. B., Steenstrup, O. R., Jonasson, J., Lindsten, J. and Zech, L.: Prenatal diagnosis of chromosome abnormalities. Acta Paediat. Scand. 61:397-404, 1972.
Case No. 91 in this report.
46,XX,t(15;19)(p1;q1).
46,XY,der(15)der(19)t(15;19)(p1;q1)mat.

Thomas, G. H.: Personal communication, 1974.
Case No. 1938 in this report.
46,XX,15p+.

Yoder, F. E., Bias, W. B., Borgaonkar, D. S., Bahr, G. F., Yoder, I. I., Yoder, O. C. and Golomb, H. M.: Cytogenetic and linkage studies of a familial 15p+ variant. Amer. J. Hum. Genet. 26:535-548, 1974.
46,XX and XY,15p+.
46,XX and XY,der(15p+)mat and pat.
Mutant Cell Repository No. GM-146.

15p110   Variable band

Niebuhr, E.:   Dicentric and monocentric Robert-

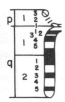

sonian translocations in man. Humangenetik 16:217-226, 1972.
Case 3 in this report.
45,XX,tdic(15;21)(p11;p13).
45,XX,tdic(15;21)(15qter to 15p11::21p13 to 21pter).

15p130   Variable band

Same entry as in 0Xq130 (Lucas and Smithies, 1974).

Same entry as in 14p120 (Rocchi, de Capoa and Gigliani, 1971).

15q000

Same entry as in 11q000 (Bochkov et al., 1974).

Same entry as in 11q000 (Breg, Schreck and Miller, 1974).

Bucher , W., Parker, C. E., Crandall, B. F. and Alfi, O. S.: Partial trisomy of chromosome 15. Lancet 1:1250, 1973.
47,X?,+del(15q-).

Dutrillaux, B.: Nouveau systeme de marquage chromosomique: Les bandes T. Chromosoma 41:395-402, 1973.
t(15q-;21q+).

Same entry as in 01q200 (Jacobs et al., 1974).

Parker, C. E. and Alfi, O. S.: Partial trisomy of chromosome 15. Lancet 1:1073, 1972.
47,XX,+15q-.

Same entry as in 02q000 (Wurster et al., 1969).

15q100

Borgaonkar, D. S., Ebenezer, L., Scott, C. I., Golomb, H. M. and Bahr, G. F.: Identification of a D/E (15/18) translocation chromosome by quinacrine fluorescence and Urea banding techniques. Humangenetik 17:317-321, 1973.
Cytogenet. Cell Genet. 12:370-371, 1973.

45,XY,-15,-18,+t(15;18) (q1;q23).
45,XY,-15,-18,+t(15;18) (18pter tc 18q23::15q1
to15qter).
Mutant Cell Repository No. GM-17.

Same entry as in 0Xq280 (Engel, Vogel and Reinwein, 1971).

Same entry as in 01p360 (Hecht, 1974).

15q110   Negative band

Same entry as in 10q110 (Hirschhorn, Lucas and
Wallace, 1973).

Hoo, J. J., Hillig, U., Cramer, M., Hansen, S.
and Hermann, F.: Familial short arm deletion of
chromosome No. 15.   Humangenetik 21:283-286,
1974.
46,XX,del(15) (q11).
46,XX,del(15) (qter to q11:).
The interpretation of a familial short arm
deletion of chromosome 15 is of interest.

Same entry as in 0Yp110 (Subrt and Blehova,
1974).

15q120   Positive band

Same entry as in 09q330 (Aula and Karjalainen,
1973).

Same entry as in 06q250 (Mikkelsen and Dyggve,
1973).

15q130   Negative band

Rethore, M. O., Dutrillaux, B. and Lejeune, J.:
Translocation 46,XX,t(15;21) (q13;q22,1) chez la
mere de deux enfants atteints de trisomie 15 et
de monosomie 21 partielles. Ann. Genet. 16:271-
275, 1973.
46,XX,t(15;21) (q13;q221).
46,XX,t(15;21) (15pter to 15q13::21q221 to
21qter;21pter to 21q221::15q13 to 15qter).
46,XX and XY,-21,+der(15)t(15;21) (q13;q221)mat.
46,XX and XY,-21,+der(15)t(15;21) (15pter to
15q13::21q221 to 21qter)mat.

15q140   Positive band

Same entry as in 01p360 (Steffensen, 1974).

15q200

Hasegawa, T., Pfeiffer, R. A., Metz, F. and Schild, W.: Balanced translocation t(15q-;16p+) as a cause of habitual abortions. Geburtshilfe Frauenheilkd 33:541-544, 1973.
46,XX,t(15;16)(q2;p1).
46,XX,t(15;16)(15pter to 15q2::16p1 to 16pter;16qter to 16p1::15q2 to 15qter).

Same entry as in 08p110 (Jacobs et al., 1974).

Laurent, C., Noel, B. and David, M.: Classification of the Dq- syndromes. Report of a 15q-patient. Ann. Genet. 14:33-40, 1971.
46,XX,del(15)(q2).
46,XX,del(15)(pter to q2:).
Chromosome identification by autoradiography.

Magenis, R. E., Overton, K. M., Reiss, J. A., MacFarlane, J. P. and Hecht, F.: Partial trisomy 15. Lancet 2:1365-1366, 1972.
47,XX,+del(15)(q2).
47,XX,+del(15)(pter to q2:).

Same entry as in 13q100 (Pasquali et al., 1973).

Webb, G. C., Garson, O. M., Robson, M. K. and Pitt, D. B.: A partial D-trisomy/normal mosaic female. J. Med. Genet. 8:522-527, 1971.
46,XX/47,XX,+del(15)(q2).
46,XX/47,XX,+del(15)(pter to q2:).

15q210   Positive band

Howard, P. N., Stoddard, G. R. and Yarbrough, K. M.: Partial trisomy D and Giemsa banding. Amer. J. Hum. Genet. 26:41A, 1974.
47,XX,+del(15)(q21).
47,XX,+del(5)(pter to q21:).

Same entry as in 02q230 (Jacobs et al., 1974).

15q220   Negative band

Fujimoto, A., Towner, J. W., Ebbin, A.J., Kahlstrom, E. J. and Wilson, M. G.: Inherited partial duplication of chromosome No. 15. J. Med. Genet. 11:287-290, 1974.
Dr. A. Fujimoto, Personal Communication, 1974.
46,XX,t(15;21)(q22;q22).
46,XY,-21,+der(21)t(15;21)(q22;q22)mat.
46,XY,-21,+der(21)t(15;21)(21pter to 21q22::15q22 to 15qter).
The offspring probably is trisomic for the region 15q22 to 15qter and monosomic for the region 21q22 to 21qter.

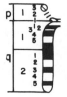

15q240   Negative band

Same entry as in 10q110 (Hirschhorn, Lucas and Wallace, 1973).

15q260   Negative band

Same entry as in 10q200 (Yunis and Sanchez, 1974).

160000

Craig-Holmes, A. P., Moore, F. B. and Shaw, M. W.: Polymorphism of human C-band heterochromatin. I. Frequency of variants. Amer. J. Hum. Genet. 25:181-192, 1974.

Machin, G. A.: Chromosome abnormality and perinatal death. Lancet 1:549-551, 1974.
46,XX,-21,+t(16p21p).

Machin, G. A. and Crolla, J. A.: Chromosome constitution of 500 infants dying during the perinatal period. Humangenetik 23:183-198, 1974.
Case No. 25 in this report.
46,XX,-21,+t(16p21p).

Same entry as in 0Y0000 (Park et al., 1974).

Same entry as in 010000 (Robson et al., 1969).

16p100

Same entry as in 15q200 (Hasegawa et al., 1973).

16p130   Negative band

    Same entry as in 01q210 (Jacobs et al., 1974).

    Same entry as in 05q200 (Jacobs et al., 1974).

16q000

    Arakaki, D. T. and Waxman, S. H.: Cytogenetics
    of spontaneous abortion. Amer. J. Obstet. Gynec.
    107:1199-1204, 1970.
    46,XX,16q+.
    47,XY,+der(16q+)mat.

    Daniel, W. L.: A genetic and biochemical inves-
    tigation of primary microcephaly. Amer. J. Ment.
    Defic. 75:653-662, 1971.
    46,XY/46,XY,16q+/46,XY,16q+,18q-.

    Same entry as in 030000 (Leisti, 1971).

    Magenis, R. E., Hecht, F. and Lovrien, E. W.:
    Heritable fragile site on chromosome 16: probable
    localization of haptoglobin locus in man.
    Science 170:85-87, 1970.

    Same entry as in 02q000 (Robson et al., 1969).

    Same entry as in 0Yq100 (Ruzicska and Czeizel,
    1970).

16q100

    Eriksson, B., Fraccaro, M., Hulten, M., Lindsten,
    J., Thoren, C. and Tiepolo, L.: Structural
    abnormalities of chromosome 18. II-   Two
    familial translocations B/18 and 16/18, ascer-
    tained through unbalanced forms. Ann. Genet.
    14:281-290, 1971.
    46,XY,t(16;18)(q1;q2).
    46,XY,der(16)der(18)t(16;18)(q1;q2)pat.
    Case No. 2 in this report.
    46,XX,-18,+der(18)t(16;18)(q1;q2)pat.
    46,XX,-18,+der(18)t(16;18)(18pter to 18q2::16q1
    to 16qter)pat.
    Meiotic studies on the father of case 2 showed a
    quadrivalent.
    Chromosome identification by autoradiography.

Mikelsaar, A. V. N., Tuur, S. J. and Kyaosaar, M.
E.: Human karyotype polymorphism. I. Routine and
fluorescence microscopic investigation of chromosomes in a normal adult population. Humangenetik
20:89-101, 1973.

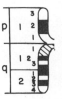

16q110   Variable band

Same entry as in 09p240 (Buckton, 1972).

Chemke, J. and Robinson, A.: The inheritance of
one chromosome No. 16 in a kindred (46,16-,C+).
J. Med. Genet. 8:346-350, 1971.
16qh+.

del Solar, C. and Uchida, I. A.: Identification
of chromosomal abnormalities by quinacrine-
staining technique in patients with normal
karyotypes by conventional analysis. J. Pediat.
84:534-538, 1974.
46,XX,inv(16)(q11q22).
46,XX,inv(16)(pter to q11::q22 to q11::q22 to
qter).
Case No. 26 in this report.
46,XY,der(16)inv(16)(q11q22)mat.

16q120   Positive band

Same entry as in 01q120 (Friedrich and Nielsen,
1974).

16q200

Same entry as in 09p200 (Alfi et al., 1973).

Francke, U.: Quinacrine mustard fluorescence of
human chromosomes: characterization of unusual
translocations. Amer. J. Hum. Genet. 24:189-213,
1972.
46,XY,t(16;22)(q2;q1).
Case No. 10: KD 071668 in this report.
46,XX,-22,+der(22)t(16;22)t(q2;q-)pat.

16q220   Negative band

Same entry as in 16q110 (del Solar and Uchida,
1974).

Same entry as in 01p320 (Jacobs et al., 1974).

16q240   Negative band

Same entry as in 01p320 (Jacobs et al., 1974).

170000

Same entry as in 110000 (Breg et al., 1972).

Same entry as in 01q420 (de la Chapelle, 1974).

Same entry as in 120000 (Machin and Crolla, 1974).

17p100

Borgaonkar, D. S. and Lewis, B. M.: Unpublished data, 1974.
Subjects No. 2186, 2187, 2188 and 2190 and Patient No. 5484 in this laboratory.
46,XY,17p+.
46,XY,der(17p+)pat.

Borgaonkar, D. S., McKusick, V. A. and Farber, P. A.: An inherited small extra chromosome. A mother with 46,XX,t(17;22)(p1;q1) and a son with 47,XY,+der(22)mat. J. Med. Genet. 10:379-383, 1973.
46,XX,t(17;22)(p1;q1).
46,XX,t(17;22)(17qter to 17p1::22q1 to 22qter;22pter to 22q1:).
47,XY,+der(22)t(17;22)(p1;q1)mat.
47,XY,+der(22)t(17;22)(22pter to 22q1:)mat.

Crandall, B. F., Carrel, R. E. and Sparkes, R. S.: Chromosome findings in 700 children referred to a psychiatric clinic. J. Pediat. 80:62-68, 1972.
Patients R.H. and D.C. in this report.
46,XY,17ps.

Same entry as in 02p100 (Dallapiccola, 1971).

Engel, E., McGee, B. J., Flexner, J. M., Russell, M. T. and Myers, B. J.: Philadelphia chromosome (Ph1) translocation in an apparently Ph1 negative, minus 22, case of chronic myeloid leukemia. New Eng. J. Med. 291:154, 1974.

45,XY,-22,+t(17;22)(p1q2;p1).
45,XY,-22,+t(17;22)(22pter to 22q1::17p1 to 17q2::22q1 to 22qter).

Kyaosaar, M. E. and Mikelsaar, A. V. N.: Chromosome investigation in married couples with repeated abortions. Humangenetik 17:277-283, 1973.
Case No. 8 in this report.
46,XY,17ps.

Leisti, J.: Structural variation in human mitotic chromosomes. Ann. Acad. Sci. fenn. (Med.) Series A, IV, Biologica 179:1-69, 1971.
Case No. 5 in this report.
46,XX,17p+.

Mikelsaar, A. V. N., Tuur, S. J. and Kyaosaar, M. E.: Human karyotype polymorphism. I. Routine and fluorescence microscopic investigation of chromosomes in a normal adult population. Humangenetik 20:89-101, 1973.

Nakagome, Y., Iinuma, K. and Matsui, I.: Three translocations involving C- or G-group chromosomes. J. Med. Genet. 10:174-176, 1973.
Case C in this report.
45,XX,-17,-22,+t(17;22)(p12 or 13;q11?)
45,XX,-17,-22,+t(17;22)(17qter to 17p12 or 13::22q11? to 22qter).

Petit, P. and Koulischer, L.: Report of a case of 46,XX/46,XX,17r mosaicism. Ann. Genet. 14:55-58, 1971.
46,XX/46,XX,r(17).
Chromosome identification by autoradiography.

Priest, J. H., Peakman, D. C., Patil, S. R. and Robinson, A.: Significance of chromosome 17ps+ in three generations of a family. J. Med. Genet. 7:142-147, 1970.

Sandstrom, M. M. and Jenkins, E. C.: A 17p marker chromosome familial study. Ann. Genet. 16:267-269, 1973.

Wikramanayake, E., Renwick, J. H. and Ferguson-Smith, M. A.: Chromosomal heteromorphisms in the

assignment of loci to particular autosomes: a study of four pedigrees. Ann. Genet. 14:245-256, 1971.
Family JN1AN in this report.
46,XY,17ps+.
46,XX and XY,der(17ps+)pat.
Propositus in this report.
46,XY,der(17ps+)pat.
The propositus was investigated for hypogonadism.

17p110   Negative band

Same entry as in 13q140 (Wilroy, Summitt and Martens, 1974).

17p130   Negative band

Same entry as in 01p320 (de la Chapelle, 1973).

Macintyre, M. N., Walden, D. B. and Hempel, J. M.: Tertiary trisomy in a human kindred containing an E/G translocation. Amer. J. Hum. Genet. 23:431-441, 1971, and personal communication, 1973.
46,XX,t(17;22)(p13;q11).
Mutant Cell Repository No. GM-119.
46,XX and XY,der(17)der(22)t(17;22)(p13;q11)mat.
Proband DP 260665 in this report.
47,XX,+der(22)t(17;22)(p13;q11)mat.

Same entry as in 10q240 (Mellman, 1974).

Same entry as in 0Xp110 (Pearson, van der Linden and Hagemeijer, 1974).

Same entry as in 13q140 (Schinzel, Schmid and Murset, 1974).

17q000

Bochkov, N. P., Kuleshov, N. P., Chebotarev, A. N., Alekhin, V. I. and Midian, S. A.: Population cytogenetic investigation of newborns in Moscow. Humangenetik 22:139-152, 1974.
46,XY,t(17q-;21q+).

Ikeuchi, T. and Fujimoto, S.: A familial transmission of heterozygous No. 17 chromosomes in

relation to spontaneous abortion. Jap. J. Hum. Genet. 43:383-387, 1968.
46,XX,17q-.
46,XX,der(17q-)mat.

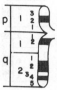

Same entry as in 13q000 (Martin, Thorburn and Smith-Read, 1970).

Same entry as in 02q000 (Masterson et al., 1970).

Same entry as in 03p000 (Subrt and Prchlikova, 1969).

17q110   Negative band

Same entry as in 11p150 (Jacobs et al., 1974).

Latta, E. and Hoo, J. J.: Trisomy of the short arm of chromosome 17. Humangenetik 23:213-217, 1974.
47,XX,+del(17)(q11).
47,XX,+del(17)(pter to q11:).

17q120   Positive band

Same entry as in 05p140 (Berger et al., 1974).

17q130   Negative band

Same entry as in 11p150 (Francke, 1974).

17q200

Same entry as in 17p100 (Engel et al., 1974).

Same entry as in 0Xp110 (Fellous, 1974).

Same entry as in 11p100 (Francke, 1972).

Same entry as in 04q200 (Jacobs et al., 1974).

Same entry as in 14q000 (Orye and van Nevel, 1968).

17q210   Negative band

Same entry as in 11p150 (Francke, 1974).

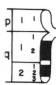

Same entry as in 01q210 (Friedrich and Nielsen, 1974).

Same entry as in 01q120 (Jacobs et al., 1974).

Same entry as in 12q240 (Machin, 1974).

17q230   Negative band

Hirschhorn, K.: Personal Communication, 1974.
46,XX,t(17;19)(q23;p13).
Mutant Cell Repository No. GM-271.

Same entry as in 03p140 (Subrt, 1974).

17q250   Negative band

Same entry as in 01q120 (Friedrich and Nielsen, 1974).

Same entry as in 02q310 (Friedrich and Nielsen, 1974).

180000

Cohen, M. M., Finch, A. B. and Lubs, H. A.:
Trisomy 18 with an E/G translocation [46,XY,21-
,t(21q18q)+]. Identification of the component
chromosomes by several laboratory techniques.
Ann. Genet. 15:45-49, 1972.
Patient J. D. in this report.
46,XY,-21,+t(18q21q).

Cohen, M. M. and Putnam, T. I.: An 18p21q
translocation in a patient with presumptive
"monosomy G." Amer. J. Dis. Child. 124:908-910,
1972.
45,XX,-18,-21,+t(18p21q).

Fraccaro, M., Herin, P., Hulten, M., Ivemark, B.
I., Jonasson, J., Lindsten, J., Tiepolo, L. and
Zetterqvist, P.: Structural abnormalities of
chromosome 18. III. Two G/18 translocations, one
identified as 22/18. Ann. Genet. 15:93-98, 1972.
Case No. 2 in this report.
45,XY,t(18q22q).

Hecht, F., Bryant, J., Arakaki, D. T., Kaplan, E.

and Gentile, G.: Trisomy-18 syndrome due to de-
novo translocation. Lancet 1:114, 1963.
46,-D,+t(Dq18q).

Same entry as in 130000 (Kistenmacher, DiGeorge
and Punnett, 1974).

Marcelli, A., Benajam, A., Poirier, J. C.,
Dansset, J., Rethore, M. O., Prieur, M. and
Lejeune, J.: A modification of the expression of
the ABO locus in a subject with karyotype
47,XY(?18q-)+. Humangenetik 22:233-241, 1974.
46,XY,t(18p20p)t,(18q20q).
46,XX,der t(18p20p),der t(18q20q)pat.
47,XY,+der t(18p20p)mat.

Muller, H., Buhler, E. M., Signer, E., Egli, F.
and Stalder, G. R.: Trisomy-18 syndrome caused
by translocation or isochromosome formation: A
case report with bibliography. J. Med. Genet.
9:462-465, 1972.
47,XX,-18,+t(18p18p),+t(18q18q) or 47,XX,-18,+
i(18p),+i(18q).

Nielsen, J., Hreidarsson, A. B., Berggreen, S.,
Ried, E., Tsuboi, T. and Saldana-Garcia, P.: A
mentally retarded male with karyotype 47,XY,+mar
- ?i(18p). Ann. Genet. 17:129-133, 1974).
47,XY,+?i(18p).

Tangheroni, W., Cao, A. and Furbetta, M.:
Multiple anomalies associated with an extra small
metacentric chromosome: modified Giemsa stain
results. Humangenetik 18:291-295, 1973.
47,XX,i(18p).
Giemsa staining technique results suggest that
the extra small metacentric chromosome is an
isochromosome for the short arm of chromosome 18.

Waldenmaier, C., Hirsch, W., Konig, E. and
Shibata, K.: Identification of a 18/21 translocation with Klinefelter's syndrome by G-band
patterns. Humangenetik 21:323-329, 1974.
47,XXY,t(18q21q).

18p110   Negative band

Same entry as in 04q000 (Bobrow and Pearson,

1971).

Borgaonkar, D. S., Bias, W. B., Scott, C. I., Wadia, R. S. and Borkowf, S. P.: IgA and abnormal chromosome 18. Lancet 1:206-207, 1969.
46,XX,r(18).
Same case reported by Borgaonkar, D. S. and Scott, C. I.: Ring chromosome 18. Birth Defects: Original Article Series V(No. 5):158-159, 1969.

Same entry as in 01q400 (Breg et al., 1972).

Same entry as in 08p000 (Buckton, 1972).

Christensen, K. R., Friedrich, U., Jacobsen, P., Jensen, K., Nielsen, J. and Tsuboi, T.: Ring chromosome 18 in mother and daughter. J. Ment. Defic. Res. 14:49-67, 1970.
46,XX,r(18).
46,XX,der(18)r(18)mat.

Cohen, M. M. and Putnam, T. I.: An 18p21q translocation in a patient with presumptive "monosomy G." Amer. J. Dis. Child. 124:908-910, 1972.
45,XX,-18,-21,+t(18;21)(p11;q).
45,XX,-18,-21,+t(18;21)(18qter to 18p11::21q to 21qter).

Cohen, M. M., Storm, D. F. and Capraro, V. J.: A ring chromosome (No. 18) in a cyclops. Clin. Genet. 3:249-252, 1972.
46,XX,r(18).

de Grouchy, J.: The 18p-, 18q- and 18r syndromes. Birth Defects: Original Article Series (V):74-87, 1969.

de Grouchy, J., Bonnette, J. and Salmon, C.: Deletion du bras court du chromosome 18. Ann. Genet. 9:19-26, 1966.
46,XX,del(18)(p11).
46,XX,del(18)(qter to p11:).

de Grouchy, J., Lamy, M., Thieffry, S., Arthuis, M. and Salmon, C.: Dysmorphic complexe avec oligophrenie: deletion des bras courts d'un

chromosome 17-18.   C. R. Acad. Sci. 256:1028-
1029, 1963.
46,XY,del(18)(p11).
46,XX,del(18)(qter to p11:).
Terminal deletion of the entire short arm was
first reported here.

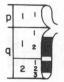

Same entry as in 09p000 (Ebbin et al., 1973).

Gilgenkrantz, S., Charles, J. M., Cabrol, C.,
Mauuary, G. and Vigneron, C.: Deletion of the
short arm of chromosome 18 due to t(22-;18p+)
with IgA deficiency. Cytogenetic study with
autoradiography and fluorescence. Ann. Genet.
15:275-281, 1972.
46,XY,t(18p+;22-).

Hecht, F. and Vlietinck, R. F.: Autosomal rings
and variable phenotypes. Humangenetik 18:99-100,
1973.
r(18).

Same entry as in 08p230 (Jacobs et al., 1974).

Kreiger, D., Palmer, C. and Biegel, A.: Human
autosomal deletion mapping and HL-A. Humangenetik 23:159-160, 1974.
46,XX,del(18)(p11).
46,XX,del(18)(qter to p11:).

Kyaosaar, M. E.:   A study of chromosomes in
couples with habitual abortions. Genetika 7:117-
121 1971 and Soviet Genetics 7:16CC-1603, 1974.
46,XX,?t(18p-;Gp+).

Same entry as in 06q210 (Klinger, 1974).

Kunze, J., Stephan, E., and Tolksdorf, M.: Ring
chromosome 18.   18p-;18q-   deletion syndrome.
Humangenetik 15:289-318. 1972.
46,XX,r(18).
A patient with ring 18 is presented and previously described cases are reviewed, and compared
with 18p-   and 18q- cases. It was concluded
that a separate 18r entity is not justifiable on
the basis of their overlapping phenotype with
18p-   and 18q- cases and suggest calling it an
18p-;18q- deletion syndrome.

Leisti, J.: Structural variation in human
mitotic chromosomes. Ann. Acad. Sci. fenn.
(Med.) Series A, IV, Biologica 179:1-69, 1971.
Case No. 17 in this report.
45,XY,t(?D-,18p+).

Lejeune, J.: Scientific impact of the study of
fine structure of chromatids. Nobel Symposium
23:16-24. 1973.
46,XX,t(18;21)(p11;q).
46,XX,t(18;21)(18qter to 18p11::21q to 2qter;21p-
ter to 21q:).
47,X?,-18,+der(18)+der(21)t(18;21)(p11;q)mat.
47,X?,-18,+der(18)+der(21)t(18;21)(18qter to
18p11::21q to 21qter;21pter to 21q:)mat.

Lubs, H. A. and Lubs, M. L.: New cytogenetic
technics applied to a series of children with
mental retardation. Nobel Symposium 23:241-250,
1973,
Patient No. 1 in this report.
46,XY,t(18;21)(p11;q11).
46,XY,t(18;21)(18qter to 18p11::21q11 to 21qter).
A karyotype previously interpreted as normal was
found to be trisomic for the long arm of chromosome 21 in a child with Down syndrome phenotype.

Lurie, J. W. and Lazjuk, G. J.: Partial monosomies 18. Review of cytogenetical and phenoty-
pical variants. Humangenetik 15:203-222. 1972.

Malpuech, G., Raynaud, E. J., Belin, J., Go-
deneche, P. and de Grouchy, J.: Short arm
deletion of chromosome 18 due to a t(21q-;18p+)
translocation. A quinacrine mustard fluorescence
analysis. Ann. Genet. 14:213-218, 1971.
46,XX,t(18;?21)(p11;q1).

Miller, J. Q., Selden, R. F. and Meisner, L. F.:
D/E translocation in a young girl. Southern Med.
J. 63:368-370, 1970.
45,XX,?t(D;18)(q;p11).
45,XX,?t(D;18)(18qter to 18p11::Dq to Dqter).

Newton, M. S., Cunningham, C., Jacobs, P. A.,
Price, W. H. and Fraser, I. A.: Chromosome
survey of a hospital for the mentally subnormal.
Part 2: Autosome abnormalities. Clin. Genet.

3:226-248, 1972.
M. R. C. Registry No. K129-192-69 in this report.
46,XY,del(18)(p11).
46,XY,del(18)(qter to p11:).

Prieur, M., Dutrillaux, B., Rethore, M. O. and
Lejeune, J.: Analyse d'une translocation t(18p+
;21q-) par denaturation menagee. Ann. Genet.
14:305-307, 1971.
46,XX,t(18p+;21q-).
47,XY,der(18)der(21)t(18p+;21q-)mat,+21.

Schinzel, A., Schmid, W., Luscher, V., Nater, M.,
Brook, C. and Steinmann, B.: Structural aberra-
tion of chromosome 18. I. The 18p- syndrome.
Arch. fur Genetik 47:1-15, 1974.
Case 1, B.C. in this report and
Case 2, K.A. in this report.
46,XX,del(18)(p11).
46,XX,del(18)(qter to p11:).
Case 3, K.F. in this report.
45,XX,-D,-18,+t(Dq18q).
A useful review of the 18p- syndrome can be
found in this report.

Summitt, R. L.: Deletion of the short arm of
chromosome 18. Cytogenetics 3:201-206, 1964.
46,XX,del(18)(p11).
46,XX,del(18)(qter to p11:).

Wertelecki, W. and Gerald, P. S.: Clinical and
chromosomal studies of the 18q- syndrome. J.
Pediat. 78:44-52, 1971.
Case No. 5 in this report.
46,XY,r(18)/46,XY,18q-.
Father of Case No. 6 in this report.
46,XY,inv(18)(pq).

Yanoff, M., Rorke, L. B. and Niederer, B. S.:
Ocular and cerebral abnormalities in chromosome
18 deletion defect. Amer. J. Ophthal. 70:391-
402, 1970.
46,XX,r(18).

18q000

Borgaonkar, D. S., Bias, W. B., Scott, C. I.,
Wadia, R. S. and Borkowf, S. P.: IgA and abnor-

mal chromosome 18.   Lancet 1:206-207, 1969.
46,XY,del(18)(q2).
46,XY,del(18)(pter to q2:).
Same case reported by Borkowf, S. P., Wadia, R.
P., Borgaonkar, D. S. and Bias, W. B.: Partial
deletion of the long arm of a chromosome 18.
Birth Defects: Original Article Series V(No.
5):155-157, 1969.

Same entry as in 01q000 (Chandley and Fletcher,
1973).

Same entry as in 16q000 (Daniel, 1971).

Same entry as in 18p110 (de Grouchy, 1969).

Same entry as in 10q000 (Dutrillaux, 1973).

Fraccaro, M., Hulten, M., Ivemark, B. I., Lindsten, J., Tiepolo, L. and Zetterqvist, P.:
Structural abnormalities of chromosome 18. I. A
case of 18q-, with autopsy findings. Ann Genet.
14:275-280, 1971.

Same entry as in 09p200 (Francke, 1972).

Same entry as in 04q000 (Hoehn, Sander and
Sander, 1971).

Same entry as in 06p000 (Jacobsen et al., 1971).

Lejeune, J., Berger, R., Rethore, M. O. and
Attal, C.:   Sur un cas, 47,XY,(?18q-)+. Ann.
Genet. 13:47-51, 1970.
46,XX,t(18q-;Fp+).
47,XY,+der(18)t(18q-;Fp+)mat.

Lubs, H. A. and Lubs, M. L.: New cytogenetic
technics applied to a series of children with
mental retardation. Nobel Symposium 23:241-250,
1973.
Patient No. 2 in this report.
46,XY,18q+.
Origin of extra segment not known.

Punnett, H. H., Pinsky, L., DiGeorge, A. M. and
Gorlin, R. J.: Familial reciprocal C/18 translocations. Amer. J. Hum. Genet. 18:572-583, 1966.

46,XX,t(C;18)(q;q).
46,XX and XY,der(C)der(18)(q;q)mat and pat.
46,XY,-18,+der(18)t(C;18)(q;q)pat.
46,XY,-18,+der(18)t(C;18)(18pter to 18q::Cq to Cqter)pat.

Same entry as in 05q000 (Rudd and Lamarche, 1971).

Same entry as in 04p100 (Schinzel and Schmid, 1972).

Same entry as in 04p100 (Schmid, 1972).

Same entry as in 09q000 (Schmid, 1972).

Subrt, I. and Pokorny, J.: Familial occurrence of 18q-. Humangenetik 10:181-187, 1970.
46,XX,18q-.
46,XX,der(18q-)mat.

Same entry as in 04q000 (Surana and Conen, 1972).

Tenbrinck, M. S.: Down's syndrome: Trisomy and translocation 47,XX,18q-,t(18q2T)+. Newport Beach, Calif., Birth Defects Conf., National Foundation - March of Dimes, p. 171, June 16-21, 1974.
47,XX,t(18q-;21),+21.

Thorburn, M. J. and Martin, P. A.: Chromosome studies in 101 mentally retarded handicapped children. J. Med. Genet. 8:59-64, 1971.
46,XY,t(C;18)(p,q).

Same entry as in 18p110 (Wertelecki and Gerald, 1971).

Yanagisawa, S.: Immunoglobulin abnormality in a girl with a large chromosome 18. J. Med. Genet. 9:360-365, 1972,
46,XX,18q+.

18q100

Same entry as in 03p100 (Breg et al., 1972).

Same entry as in 110000 (Breg et al., 1972).

Same entry as in 04q300 (Chesler et al., 1970).

Eriksson, B., Fraccaro, M., Hulten, M., Lindsten, J., Thoren, C. and Tiepolo, L.: Structural abnormalities of chromosome 18. II. Two familial translocations, B/18 and 16/18, ascertained through unbalanced forms. Ann. Genet. 14:281-290, 1971.
46,XX and XY,t(B;18)(q;q1).
46,XX and XY,t(B;18)(Bpter to Bq::18q1 to 18qter;18pter to 18q1::Bq to Bqter).
46,XX and XY,der(B)der(18)t(B;18)(q;q1)pat.
Case 1 in this report.
46,XY,-B,+der(B)t(B;18)(q;q1)pat.
46,XY,-B,+der(B)t(B;18)(Bpter to Bq::18q1 to 18qter)pat.
Chromosome identification by autoradiography.

Same entry as in 06q200 (Nakagome, Iinuma and Matsui, 1973).

Same entry as in 0Xp200 (Thelen, Abrams and Fisch, 1971).

Uchida, I. A., Wang, H. C., Laxdal, O. E., Zaleski, W. A. and Duncan, B. P.: Partial trisomy-deficiency syndrome resulting from a reciprocal translocation in a large kindred. Cytogenetics 3:81-96, 1964.
46,XX and XY,t(18;G)(q1;q).
46,XX and XY,t(18;G)(18pter to 18q1::Gq to Gqter;Gpter to Gq::18q1 to 18qter).
46,XX and XY,der(18)der(G)t(18;G)(q1;q)mat and pat.
Cases 1, 2 and 3 in this report.
46,XY,-G,+der(18)t(18;G)(q1;q)mat and pat.
46,XY,-G,+der(18)t(18;G)(18pter to 18q1::Gq to Gqter)mat and pat.

18q110   Negative band

Same entry as in 04p140 (Jacobs et al., 1974).

Lozzio, C. B. and Klepper, M. B.: Chromosome aberrations identified by the new banding techniques. Amer. J. Hum. Genet. 26:55A, 1974.
t(18;21)(q11;q22)mat.
This familial reciprocal translocation is re-

ported here.

Same entry as in 11p150 (McAlpine et al., 1974).

18q120   Positive band

Boue, J. and Boue, A.: L'interet en diagnostic prenatal des techniques nouvelles d'identification chromosomique dans des translocations et une aneusomie de recombinaison. Nouv. Presse Med. 2:3097-3102, 1973.
Observation No. 2088 in this report.
46,XX,t(18;20)(q12;p13).

Same entry as in 06p220 (Gouw, ten Kate and Anders, 1973).

18q200

Breibert, S., Mellman, W. J. and Eberlein, W. R.: Developmental retardation associated with an unbalanced 13/15/18 translocation. Cytogenetics 3:252-257, 1964.
45,XY,-D,tan(D;18)(q1;q2).

Same entry as in 16q100 (Eriksson et al., 1971).

Same entry as in 02q300 (Grosse and Schwanitz, 1973).

Same entry as in 04p100 (Jacobs et al., 1974).

Same entry as in 13q000 (McGilvray et al., 1971).

Same entry as in 04p100 (Schinzel and Schmid, 1972).

Wyandt, H. E., Hecht, F., Lovrien, E. W. and Stewart, R. E.: Study of a patient with apparent monosomy 21 owing to translocation: 45,XX,21-,t(18q+). Cytogenetics 10:413-426, 1971.
45,XX,-18,-21,+t(18;21)(q2;q).
45,XX,-18,-21,+t(18;21)(18pter to 18q2::21q to 21qter).
The patient had dyschondrosteosis and mild mental retardation.

Wyandt, H. E., Vlietinck, R. F., Magenis, R. E.

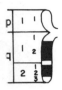

and Hecht, F.: Colored reverse-banding of human chromosomes with acridine orange following alkaline-formalin treatment: densitometric validations and applications. Humangenetik 23:119-130, 1974.
Case No. 4 in this report.
46,XY,t(18;20)(q2;q13).

18q210   Negative band

Same entry as in 01q320 (Chandley et al., 1972).

Same entry as in 09p220 (Hamerton, Ray and Douglas, 1973).

Same entry as in 01q320 (Jacobs et al., 1974).

Same entry as in 04q270 (Knorr-Gartner, Knorr and Haas, 1974).

Same entry as in 11p150 (McAlpine et al., 1974).

18q220   Positive band

Jenkins, E. C., Weed, R. G. and Sandstrom, M. M.: An additional case of partial trisomy 18. Ann. Genet. 17:45-48, 1974.
46,XY,dup(18)(q22).
46,XY,dup(18)(pter to q22::q22 to qter).

Kreiger, D., Palmer, C. and Biegel, A.: Human autosomal deletion mapping and HL-A. Humangenetik 23:159-160, 1974.
46,XX,del(18)(q22).
46,XX,del(18)(pter to q22:).

Same entry as in 01q300 (Seabright, 1972).

18q230   Negative band

Same entry as in 15q100 (Borgaonkar et al., 1973).

Same entry as in 07q320 (Thompson and Palmer, 1974).

190000

Same entry as in 14q100 (Fryns, Cassiman and van
den Berghe, 1974).

Same entry as in 0Xq200 (Gerald, 1974).

Vogel, W. and Loning, B.: Identification of a
familial 19/21 translocation by Q and G band
patterns. Humangenetik 18:219-224, 1973.
46,XX,t(19;21)(p or q13;q22).
46,XX and XY,der(19)der(21)t(19;21)(p or
q13;q22)mat.
47,XY,+21,der(19)der(21)t(19;21)(p or
q13;q22)mat.

19p100

Genest, P., Bouchard, M. and Poty, J.: Partial
deletion of a group-F(19-20) chromosome in a
physically handicapped psychiatric male patient.
J. Med. Genet. 8:374-377, 1971.
46,XY,del(19)(p1).
46,XY,del(19)(qter to p1:).
Chromosome identification by autoradiography.

Newton, M. S., Cunningham, C., Jacobs, P. A.,
Price, W. H. and Fraser, I. A.: Chromosome
survey of a hospital for the mentally subnormal.
Part 2: Autosome abnormalities. Clin. Genet.
3:226-248, 1972.
M. R. C. Registry No. K175-17-67 in this report.
46,XY,t(19p-;22q+).

Uchida, I. A. and Lin, C. C.: Ring formation of
chromosomes Nos. 19 and 20. Cytogenetics 11:208-
215, 1972.
Case 1, H.W. in this report.
46,XX,/46,XX,r(19).

19p130   Negative band

Hamerton, J. L., Ray, M. and Douglas, G. R.:
Chromosome banding techniques in clinical cytogenetics. Nobel Symposium 23:203-213, 1973.
Case No. AC090472, NB-8732.01 in this report.
46,XX,inv(19)(p13q13).
46,XX,inv(19)(pter to p13::q13 to p13::q13 to
qter).
Case No. AC090472, NB-8732 in this report.

47,XY,der(19)inv(19)(p13q13)mat,+21.

Same entry as in 17q230 (Hirschhorn, 1974).

Jacobs, P. A., Buckton, K. E., Cunningham, C. and Newton, M. S.: An analysis of the break points of structural rearrangements in man. J. Med. Genet. 11:50-64, 1974.
M. R. C. Registry No. K82-54-70 in this report.
46,XY,inv(19)(p13q12 or 13).
46,XY,inv(19)(pter to p13::q12 or 13 to p13::q12 or 13 to qter.).

Same entry as in 03p110 (Jacobs et al., 1974).

Same entry as in 06p250 (Pallister et al., 1974).

Same entry as in 09p100 (Rethore et al., 1970).

Sekhon, G. S., Hillman, L. S. and Kaufman, R. L.: Identification of a 19/20 translocation by G, Q and C banding. Newport Beach Calif., Birth Defects Conf., National Foundation - March of Dimes, p. 92, June 16-21, 1974.
46,XX,t(19;20)(p13;p13).

19q100

Same entry as in 22q100 (Gahrton, Zech and Lindsten, 1974).

Same entry as in 19p130 (Jacobs et al., 1974).

Same entry as in 07q000 (Newton et al., 1972).

Same entry as in 15p100 (Therkelsen et al., 1972).

19q130   Negative band

Same entry as in 07q320 (Buckton 1972).

Same entry as in 09q210 (Friedrich and Nielsen, 1974).

Same entry as in 19p130 (Hamerton, Ray and Douglas, 1973).

Jacobs, P. A., Buckton, K. E., Cunningham, C. and
Newton, M. S.: An analysis of the break points
in structural rearrangements in man. J. Med.
Genet. 11:50-64, 1974.
M. R. C. Registry No. K175-17-67 in this report.
46,XY,t(19;22)(q13;q13).

Same entry as in 11q140 (Jacobs et al., 1974).

200000

Same entry as in 180000 (Marcelli et al., 1974).

20p100

Same entry as in 06q210 (Allderdice et al.,
1971).

Atkins, L., Miller, W. L. and Salam, M.: A ring-
20 chromosome. J. Med. Genet. 9:377-380, 1972.
46,XX,r(20).

Same entry as in 13q300 (Francke, 1972).

Uchida, I. A. and Lin, C. C.: Ring formation of
chromosomes Nos. 19 and 20. Cytogenetics 11:208-
215, 1972.
Case 2, S. C. in this report.
46,XX/46,XX,r(20).

20p110   Negative band

Same entry as in 03q290 (Jacobs et al., 1974).

Subrt, I. and Brychnac, V.: Trisomy for the
short arm of chromosome 20. Humangenetik 23:219-
222, 1974.
46,XX,t(20;21)(p11;p11).
46,XX,t(20;21)(20pter to 20p11::21p11 to
21qter;21pter to 21p11::20p11 to 20qter).
46,XX,-21,+der(21)t(20;21)(p11;p11)mat.
46,XX,-21,+der(21)t(20;21)(20pter to 20p11::21p11
to 21qter)mat.

20p130   Negative band

Same entry as in 18q120 (Boue and Boue, 1973).

Same entry as in 11q130 (Hamerton, Ray and Douglas, 1973).

Same entry as in 19p130 (Sekhon, Hillman and Kaufman, 1974).

20q100

Same entry as in 04q200 (Francke, 1972).

Same entry as in 14q000 (Krompotic et al., 1971).

20q110   Negative band

Same entry as in 14p110 (Kreiger, Palmer and Biegel, 1974).

20q130   Negative band

Same entry as in 14q220 (Fawcett, McCord and Francke, 1974).

Same entry as in 18q200 (Wyandt et al., 1974).

210000

Same entry as in 140000 (Boue and Boue, 1973).

Same entry as in 140000 (Caspersson et al., 1971).

Same entry as in 130000 (Caspersson et al., 1971).

Caspersson, T., Hulten, M., Lindsten, J., Therke-lsen, A. J. and Zech, L.: Identification of different Robertsonian translocations in man by quinacrine mustard fluorescence analysis.
Hereditas 67:213-220, 1971.
Cases 8, 10 and 11 in this report.
45,XX,t(21q21q).
Case 9 in this report.
45,XX,t(21q22q).

Same entry as in 180000 (Cohen, Finch and Lubs, 1972).

Same entry as in 180000 (Cohen and Putnam, 1972).

Same entry as in 140000 (Chrz, Kczak and Malkova, 1973).

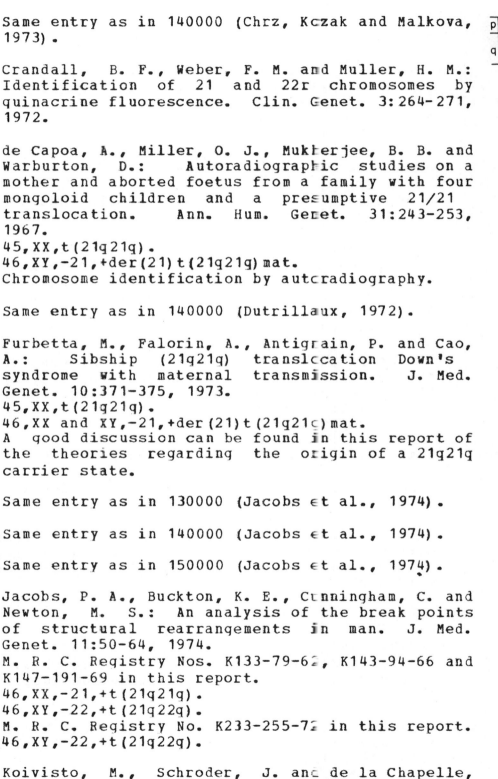

Crandall, B. F., Weber, F. M. and Muller, H. M.: Identification of 21 and 22r chromosomes by quinacrine fluorescence. Clin. Genet. 3:264-271, 1972.

de Capoa, A., Miller, O. J., Mukterjee, B. B. and Warburton, D.: Autoradiographic studies on a mother and aborted foetus from a family with four mongoloid children and a presumptive 21/21 translocation. Ann. Hum. Genet. 31:243-253, 1967.
45,XX,t(21q21q).
46,XY,-21,+der(21)t(21q21q)mat.
Chromosome identification by autcradiography.

Same entry as in 140000 (Dutrillaux, 1972).

Furbetta, M., Falorin, A., Antigrain, P. and Cao, A.: Sibship (21q21q) translccation Down's syndrome with maternal transmission. J. Med. Genet. 10:371-375, 1973.
45,XX,t(21q21q).
46,XX and XY,-21,+der(21)t(21q21c)mat.
A good discussion can be found in this report of the theories regarding the origin of a 21q21q carrier state.

Same entry as in 130000 (Jacobs et al., 1974).

Same entry as in 140000 (Jacobs et al., 1974).

Same entry as in 150000 (Jacobs et al., 1974).

Jacobs, P. A., Buckton, K. E., Cunningham, C. and Newton, M. S.: An analysis of the break points of structural rearrangements in man. J. Med. Genet. 11:50-64, 1974.
M. R. C. Registry Nos. K133-79-62, K143-94-66 and K147-191-69 in this report.
46,XX,-21,+t(21q21q).
46,XY,-22,+t(21q22q).
M. R. C. Registry No. K233-255-72 in this report.
46,XY,-22,+t(21q22q).

Koivisto, M., Schroder, J. anc de la Chapelle,

A.: Probable monosomy-21 and partial trisomy. Amer. J. Dis. Child. 125:426-428, 1973.

Lucas, M. and Wallace, I.: Recurrent abortions and chromosome abnormalities. J. Obstet. Gynaec. Brit. Comm. 79:1119-1127, 1972.
Family Gi in this report.
46,XY,-21,+t(21q21q).

Same entry as in 160000 (Machin, 1974).

Same entry as in 160000 (Machin and Crolla, 1974).

Mathew, E. B., Dietzman, D. E., Madden, D. L., Sever, J. L., Al-Aish, M. S. and Dodson, E. D.: Possible absence of Australian antigen in G/G translocation-type Down's syndrome. Lancet 1:702, 1971.
46,?,-21,+t(21q21q).

Shibata, K., Waldenmaier, C. and Hirsch, W.: A child with a 21 ring chromosome, 45,XX,21-/ 46,XX,21r. Investigated with banding technique. Humangenetik 18:315-319, 1973.
45,XX,-21/46,XX,r(21).

Same entry as in 18q000 (Tenbrinck, 1974).

Same entry as in 180000 (Waldenmaier et al., 1974).

Yang, S. J. and Rosenberg, H. S.: 21-22 translocation Down's syndrome: A family with unusual segregating patterns. Amer. J. Hum. Genet. 21:248-251, 1969.

21p100

Atkins, L. and Feingold, M.: Case reports 46,XY,21qi/46,XY,21p-/mosaicism in a child with Down's syndrome. J. Med. Genet. 6:206-208, 1969.
46,XY,i(22q)/46,XY,21p-.

Aula, P. and Karjalainen, O.: Prenatal karyotype analysis in high risk families. Ann. Clin. Res. 5:142-148, 1973.
46,XX,t(21;22)(p1;q1).

Case No. 1 in this report.
46,XY,der(21)der(22)t(21;22)(p1;q1)mat.

de Grouchy, J.:   21p-   maternel en double exemplaire chez un trisomique 21. Ann. Genet. 13:52-55, 1970.
46,XX,21p-.
47,XX,der(21p-)mat,+der(21p-)mat.

Same entry as in 14p110 (Jacobs et al., 1974).

Kucerova, M. and Polivkova, Z.:   A case of a girl with a 21 ring chromosome. Hum. Hered. 24:100-104, 1974.
46,XX,r(21).

Magenis, R. E., Armendares, S., Hecht, F., Weber, R. G. and Overton, K.: Identification by fluorescence of two G rings: (46,XY,21r) G deletion syndrome I and (46,XX,22r) G deletion syndrome II. Ann. Genet. 15:265-266, 1972.
Patient 1 in this report.
46,XY,r(21).

Mikelsaar, A. V. N., Tuur, S. J. and Kyaosaar, M. E.: Human karyotype polymorphism. I. Routine and fluorescence microscopic investigation of chromosomes in a normal adult population. Humangenetik 20:89-101, 1973.

Monteleone, P. L., Monteleone, J. A., Rivard, D. and Grzegocki, J. A.: Elongated short arm of a G-group chromosome associated with similar phenotypic abnormalities in three patients. J. Pediat. 83:473-476, 1973.
Patients 1, 2 and 3 in this report.
46,XY,21p+.

Nielsen, J., Friedrich, U. and Hreidarsson, A. B.:   Frequency of deletion of short arm satellites in acrocentric chromosomes. J. Med. Genet. 11:177-180, 1974.
46,XX,22ps-.
Propositus No. 7353 in this report.
46,XY,der(22ps-)mat.

Same entry as in 05p100 (Singer and Scaife, 1970).

Same entry as in 0Xq110 (Summitt, Martens and Wilroy, 1974).

Warren, R. J., Rimoin, D. L. and Summitt, R. L.: Identification by fluorescent microscopy of the abnormal chromosomes associated with the G-deletion syndromes. Amer. J. Hum. Genet. 25:77-81, 1973.
Case 1 in this report.
46,XY,r(21).
Partial deletion of the long arm, as well as a ring chromosome 21, results, according to these authors and others, in a characteristic pheno-type, called G I deletion syndrome.

21p110   Variable band

Borgaonkar, D. S. and Mules, E.: Unpublished observation, 1974.
Patient No. 5772 in this laboratory.
46,XX,del(21)(p11).
46,XX,del(21)(qter to p11:).

Cantu, J. M., Salamanca, F., Sanchez, J., Pena, T., Pacheco, C. and Armendares, S.: Human acrocentric rings and "satellite" association. Amer. J. Hum. Genet. 26:18A, 1974.
Case B in this report.
46,XY,r(21)(p11q22).
Case D in this report.
46,XY/47,XY,+r(21)(p11q22).

Kreiger, D., Palmer, C. and Biegel, A.: Human autosomal deletion mapping and HL-A. Humangene-tik 23:159-160, 1974.
46,XY,-21,+t(21;21)(p11;p11).

Niebuhr, E.: Dicentric and monocentric Robert-sonian translocations in man. Humangenetik 16:217-226, 1972.
Case 5 in this report.
45,XY,tdic(21;22)(p11;p12).
45,XY,tdic(21;22)(21qter to 21p11::22p12 to 22qter).

Same entry as in 20p110 (Subrt and Brychnac, 1974).

21p120   Variable band

Hillman, L. S., Sekhon, G. S., Kaufman, R. L. and
Ho, C. K.: Y/21 translocation with gonadal and
renal dysgenesis and cardiac rupture. Amer. J.
Dis. Child. 128:560-563, 1974.
46,X,-21,+t(Y;21)(q121;p12).
46,X,-21,+t(Y;21)(21qter to 21p12::Yq121 to
Yqter).

Same entry as in 04p110 (Seabright, 1974).

21p130   Variable band

Cantu, J. M., Salamanca, F., Sanchez, J., Pena,
T., Pacheco, C. and Armendares, S.:   Human
acrocentric rings and "satellite" association.
Amer. J. Hum. Genet. 26:18A, 1974.
Case A in this report.
46,XY,r(21)(p13q22).

Hirschhorn, K., Lucas, M. and Wallace, I.:
Precise identification of various chromosomal
abnormalities.   Ann. Hum. Genet. 36:375-379,
1973.
Family Gi(GC686) in this report.
45,XY,t(21:21)(p13;q21).
45,XY,t(21;21)(21qter to 21p13::21q21 to 21qter).
46,XY,-21,+der(21)t(21;21)(p13;q21)pat.

Same entry as in 15p110 (Niebuhr, 1972).

Uchida, I. A.:   Paternal origin of the extra
chromosome in Down's syndrome. Lancet 2:1258,
1973.
Two brightly satellited No. 21 chromosomes in a
Down syndrome patient were found to be of paternal origin.

Same entry as in 07q310 (Vogel, Siebers and
Reinwein, 1973).

21q000

Same entry as in 17q000 (Bochkov et al., 1974).

Same entry as in 18p110 (Cohen and Putnam, 1972).

Cohen, M. M. and Davidson, R. G.: Down's syndrome associated with a familial (21q-;22q+) translocation. Cytogenetics 6:321-330, 1967.
46,XX,t(21;22)(q;q13).
46,XX and XY,der(21)der(22)t(21;22)(q;q13)mat.
Cases 1 and 2 in this report.
46,XX and XY,-22,+der(22)t(21;22)(q;q13)mat.
46,XX and XY,-22,+der(22)t(21;22)(22pter to 22q13::21q to 21qter)mat.

Same entry as in 05p100 (DeGeorge, Neu and Gardner, 1974).

Same entry as in 15q000 (Dutrillaux, 1973).

Same entry as in 10q200 (Francke, 1972).

Same entry as in 010000 (Kontras et al., 1966).

Same entry as in 18p110 (Lejeune, 1973).

Same entry as in 18p110 (Prieur et al., 1971).

Same entry as in 13q000 (Talvik et al., 1973).

Same entry as in 02q000 (Wahrman et al., 1974).

Same entry as in 18q200 (Wyandt et al., 1971).

21q110   Negative band

Bartsch-Sandhoff, M. and Schade, H.: Two subterminal heterochromatin regions in a rare form of 21/21 translocation. Humangenetik 18:329-336, 1973.
46,XX,tan(21;21).

Same entry as in 06p250 (Borgaonkar et al., 1973).

Hongell, K. and Airaksinen, E.: A Gq deletion in a girl with Down's syndrome. Hum. Hered. 22:80-85, 1972.
47,XX,del(21)(q11)/47,XX,+21.
47,XX,del(21)(pter to q11:)/47,XX,+21.

Same entry as in 18p110 (Lubs and Lubs, 1973).

Vogel, W.: Identification of G-group chromosomes involved in a G/G tandem-translocation by the Giemsa-band technique. Humangenetik 14:255-256, 1972.
46,XY,tan(21;21)(q23;q11).
46,XY,tan(21;21)(21pter to 21q22::21q11 to 21qter).

21q200

Same entry as in 07q300 (Bass, Crandall and Marcy, 1973).

Finley, S. C., Finley, W. H., Rosecrans, C. J. and Phillips, C.: Exceptional intelligence in a mongoloid child of a family with a 13/15/partial 21 (D/partial G) translocation. New Eng. J. Med. 272:1089-1092, 1965.
46,XY,t(D;21)(p1;q2).
46,XX,der(D)der(21)t(D;21)(p1;q2)pat.
46,XX,-D,+der(D)t(D;21)(p1;q2)mat.

Same entry as in 07q000 (Giraud et al., 1974).

Jernigan, D., Curl, N. and Keeler, C.: Milledgeville mongoloid: A rare karyotype of Down's syndrome. J. Hered. 65:254-257, 1974.
46,XY,-21,+t(21;21)(q2;q1).
This variant tandem translocation carrier patient is called 'Milledgeville mongoloid'.

Same entry as in 02p100 (Miller et al., 1970).

Same entry as in 09p200 (Rethore et al., 1972).

Same entry as in 13q000 (Talvik et al., 1973).

21q210   Positive band

Same entry as in 21p130 (Cantu et al., 1974; Cases A, B and D).

Same entry as in 04q210 (de la Chapelle, Koivisto and Schroder, 1973).

Same entry as in 21p130 (Hirschhorn, Lucas and Wallace, 1973).

21q220   Negative band

Same entry as in 04q350 (Dutrillaux et al., 1973).

Same entry as in 15q220 (Fujimoto et al., 1974).

Same entry as in 11q230 (Jacobsen et al., 1973).

Same entry as in 14q120 (Laurent et al., 1973).

Same entry as in 18q110 (Lozzio and Klepper, 1974).

Same entry as in 12q140 (Mikkelsen, 1974).

Niebuhr, E.: Down's syndrome. The possibility of a pathogenetic segment on chromosome 21. Human-genetik 21:99-101, 1974.
"This paper contains a brief survey of twelve patients with a G/G translocation in tandem and it is suggested that trisomy of the band 21q22 might be pathogenetic in Down's syndrome."

Same entry as in 14q200 (Pfeiffer, Buttinghaus and Struck, 1973).

Same entry as in 08q220 (Sakurai et al., 1974).

Turk, K. B., Martin, A. O. and Macintyre, M. N.: An unusual chromosome in a child with some features of mongolism. Amer. J. Hum. Genet. 26:87A, 1974.
46,XX,t(21;21(q22;q22).
46,XX,t(21;21)(21pter to 21q22::21q22 to 21cen?).

Same entry as in 190000 (Vogel and Loning, 1973).

Same entry as in 21q110 (Vogel, 1972).

21q221   Negative band

Same entry as in 15q130 (Rethore, Dutrillaux and Lejeune, 1973).

220000

Same entry as in 210000 (Caspersson et al.,

1971).

Crandall, B. F., Weber, F., Müller, H. M. and Burwell, J. K.: Identification of 21r and 22r chromosomes by quinacrine fluorescence. Clin. Genet. 3:264-270, 1972.
Case No. 2 (AK 100751) and Case Nc. 3 (MR 211159) in this report.
46,XY,r(22).

Same entry as in 180000 (Fraccaro et al., 1972).

Same entry as in 0Yq100 (Friedrich and Nielsen, 1972).

Same entry as in 150000 (Friedrich, Nielsen and Sehested, 1972).

Same entry as in 18p110 (Gilgenkrantz et al., 1972).

Same entry as in 130000 (Jacobs et al., 1974).

Same entry as in 140000 (Jacobs et al., 1974).

Same entry as in 150000 (Jacobs et al., 1974).

Same entry as in 210000 (Jacobs et al., 1974).

Same entry as in 140000 (Lubs and Ruddle, 1970).

Same entry as in 140000 (Neu, Valentine and Gardner, 1974).

22p100   Variable band

Same entry as in 09q120 (Buckton, 1972).

Same entry as in 09q120 (Chandley et al., 1972).

Elmore, S. M., Nance, W. E., McGee, B. J., Engel de Montmollin, M. and Engel, E.: Pycnodysostosis, with a familial chromosome anomaly. Amer. J. Med. 40:273-282, 1966.
46,XY,?22p-.
46,XX and XY,der(?22p-)pat.

Same entry as in 09q100 (Evans, Buckton and

Sumner, 1971).

Fitzgerald, P. H. and Hamer, J. W.: Third case of chronic lymphocytic leukaemia in a carrier of the inherited Ch1 chromosome. Brit. Med. J. 3:752-754, 1969.
46,XX and XY,22p-.
46,XX and XY,der(22p-)mat and pat.
The Ch1 (Christchurch 1) is believed to be a G2 autosome, from which the short arm is absent.

Same entry as in 01p000 (Francke, 1972).

Same entry as in 10q200 (Francke, 1972).

Same entry as in 0Yq100 (Friedrich and Nielsen, 1972).

Hasen, J. and Bartalos, M.: Oligospermia and infertility in a man with varigocele and G chromosome translocation. J. Urol. 3:85-87, 1974.
46,XY,22p+.
The patient is thought to have a partial trisomy for an unknown chromosome segment.

Hoefnagel, D., Schroeder, T. M. and Benirschke, K.: A child with a group-G ring chromosome. Humangenetik 4:52-58, 1967.
46,XX,?22r.

Kaijser, K.: Heart malformations in two brothers with identical chromosome aberrations (46,XY,G-?F+). Clin. Genet. 2:255-260, 1971.

Lindenbaum, R. H., Bobrow, M. and Barber, L.: Monozygotic twins with ring chromosome 22. J. Med. Genet. 10:85-89, 1973.
46,XX,22(r).

Magenis, R. E., Armendares, S., Hecht, F., Weleber, R. G. and Overton, K. M.: Identification by fluorescence of two G rings: (46,XY,21r) G deletion syndrome I and (46,XX,22r) G deletion syndrome II. Ann. Genet. 15:265-266, 1972.
Patient No. 2 in this report.
46,XX,22(r).

Same entry as in 04p100 (Metz, Bier and Pfeiffer, 1973).

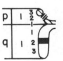

Mikelsaar, A. V. N., Tuur, S. J. and Kyaosaar, M. E.: Human karyotype polymorphism. I. Routine and fluorescence microscopic investigation of chromosomes in a normal adult population. Humangenetik 20:89-101, 1973.

Same entry as in 09q000 (Newton et al., 1972).

Same entry as in 05p140 (Niebuhr, 1972).

Nielsen, J., Friedrich, U. and Hreidarsson, H. B.: Frequency of deletion of short arm satellites in acrocentric chromosomes. J. Med. Genet. 11:177-180, 1974.
46,XY,22ps-.
Propositus No. 9995 in this report.
46,XY,der(22ps-)pat.

Nielsen, J., Friedrich, U., Hreidarsson, A. B., Noel, B., Quack, B. and Mottet, J.: Brilliantly fluorescing enlarged short arms D or G. Lancet 1:1049-1050, 1974.

Same entry as in 0Yq100 (Reitalu, 1973).

Same entry as in 09p100 (Rethore et al., 1970).

Same entry as in 08p100 (Rosenthal et al., 1973).

Stoll, C., Rohmer, A. and Sauvage, P.: 22-ring chromosome: identification by controlled heating. Ann. Genet. 16:193-198, 1973.
45,XX,-22/46,XX,r(22).

Warren, R. J., Rimoin, D. L. and Summitt, R. L.: Identification by fluorescent microscopy of the abnormal chromosomes associated with the G-deletion syndromes. Amer. J. Hum. Genet. 25:77-81, 1973.
Cases 2 and 3 in this report.
46,XX and XY,r(22).
Partial deletion of the long arm, as well as a ring chromosome 22, results, according to these authors and others, in a characteristic phenotype, called G II deletion syndrome.

Same entry as in 09p000 (Weber, Muller and Sparkes, 1974).

Whang-Peng, J., Knutsen, T. A. and Lee, E. C.: Dicentric Ph1 chromosome. J. Nat. Cancer Inst. 51:2009-2012, 1973.
A dicentric Ph1 chromosome in a single and double dose has been reported in three of the five patients.

22p110   Variable band

Same entry as in 08q220 (Lejeune et al., 1972).

Same entry as in 04p140 (Schwanitz and Grosse, 1973).

22p120   Variable band

Same entry as in 10q240 (Boue and Boue, 1973).

Same entry as in 04p110 (Giovannelli, Forabosco and Dutrillaux, 1974).

Same entry as in 04p110 (Giovannelli, Rossi and Forabosco, 1973).

Same entry as in 0Yq122 (Lundsten and Philip, 1973).

Same entry as in 21p110 (Niebuhr, 1972).

Same entry as in 10q240 (Roux, Taillemite and Baheux-Morlier, 1974).

22q100

Same entry as in 21p100 (Atkins and Feingold, 1969).

Same entry as in 21p100 (Aula and Karjalainen, 1973).

Borgaonkar, D. S.:   Philadelphia-chromosome translocation and chronic myeloid leukaemia. Lancet 1:1250, 1973.
It is suggested that the relation of Ph1 chromo-some to chronic myeloid leukemia could be that it

is a position effect phenomena. If this is borne
out to be true then it would be the first such
example in man and also first such relationship
to neoplasia.

Same entry as in 17p100 (Borgaonkar, McKusick and
Farber, 1973).

Buhler, E. M., Mehes, K., Muller, H. and Stalder,
G. R.: Cat eye syndrome, a partial trisomy 22.
Humangenetik 15:150-152, 1972.
46,XX,22q-.
46,XX,der(22q-)mat.
47,XX,+der(22q-)mat.
46,XX,der(22q-)mat/47,XX,+der(22q-)mat.

Caspersson, T., Gahrton, G., Lindsten, J. and
Zech, L.: Identification of the Philadelphia
chromosome as a number 22 by quinacrine mustard
fluorescence analysis. Exp. Cell Res. 63:238-
240, 1970.

Same entry as in 04q000 (Centerwall et al.,
1974).

Same entry as in 11q200 (Dutrillaux, 1972).

Same entry as in 17p100 (Engel et al., 1974).

Same entry as in 16q200 (Francke, 1972).

Gahrton, G., Zech, L. and Lindsten, J.: A new
variant translocation (19q+,22q-) in chronic
myelocytic leukemia. Exp. Cell Res. 86:214-216,
1974.
Patient No. 1 in this report.
46,XX,t(19q+;22q-).
Patients No. 2 to 9 in this report.
46,XX or XY,t(9q+;22q-).
See Rowley (1973) in entry 22q100.

Hayata, I., Kakati, S. and Sandberg, A. A.: A
new translocation related to the Philadelphia
chromosome. Lancet 2:1385, 1973.
46,XY,t(2;22)(q3;q1).
46,XY,t(2;22)(2pter to 2q3::22q1 to 22qter;22pter
to 22q1).
See Rowley (1973) in entry 22q100.

Same entry as in 09q000 (Lejeune, 1973).

Same entry as in 17p100 (Nakagome, Iinuma and Matsui, 1973).

Nelson, R.: Long arm deletion of chromosome 22, with protein-losing enteropathy. Proc. Roy. Soc. Med. 65:1081-1083, 1972.
46,XY,22q-.

Same entry as in 19p100 (Newton et al., 1972).

Rowley, J. D.: A new consistent chromosomal abnormality in chronic myelogenous leukaemia identified by quinacrine fluorescence and Giemsa staining. Nature 243:290-293, 1973.
46,XY,t(9;22)(q3;q1).
46,XY,t(9;22)(9pter to 9q3::22q1 to 22qter;22pter to 22q1).
It was first pointed out in this report that the Philadelphia chromosome is the result of a translocation and not a deletion, as had been thought.
For uniformity all primary reports of Philadelphia translocation are entered here after a consultation with Dr. Rowley.
See Borgaonkar (1973) in entry 22q100.

Same entry as in 01q000 (Therkelsen et al., 1972).

Same entry as in 130000 (Wennstrom and Schroder, 1973).

22q110   Negative band

Same entry as in 09q210 (Buckton, 1972).

Same entry as in 09q210 (Hirschhorn, Lucas and Wallace, 1973).

Same entry as in 17p130 (Macintyre, Walden and Hempel, 1971).

Same entry as in 08q241 (Sanchez and Yunis, 1974).

van den Berghe, H.: Personal Communication,

1974.
Brilliant Q positive band at this region.

22q120   Positive band

Foerster, W., Medan, H. J. and Loffler, H.:
Chronic granulocytic leukemia with Philadelphia-
chromosome and tandem-translocation on the second
chromosome 22;46,XX,tan(22q+;22q-). Klin. Wschr.
52: 123-126, 1974.
46,XX,tan(22;22)(q13;q12).
46,XX,tan(22;22)(22pter to 22q13::22q12 to
22qter;22pter to 22q12).
See Rowley (1973) in entry 22q100.

Same entry as in 09q340 (Whang-Peng, Lee and
Knutsen, 1974).

22q130   Negative band

Alfi, O. S., Sanger, R. G. and Donnell, G. N.:
Trisomy 22: A clinically identifiable phenotype.
Newport Beach, Calif., Birth Defects Conf.,
National Foundation -   March of Dimes, p. 93,
June 16-21, 1974.
47,XXX,del(22)(q13:).
47,XXX,del(22)(pter to q13:).
47,XXX,+der(22)del(22)(q13)mat.

Same entry as in 0Xq220 (Brown, Shows and Palmer,
1974).

Same entry as in 21q000 (Cohen and Davidson,
1967).

Same entry as in 22q120 (Foerster, Medan and
Loffler, 1974).

Same entry as in 19q130 (Jacobs et al., 1974).

Same entry as in 0Xq230 (Pearson, van der Linden
and Hagemeijer, 1974).

Same entry as in 09q100 (Rethore et al., 1970).

0X0000

Baranovskaya, L. I. and Zakharov, A. F.: H3-

deoxycytidine incorporation into X-chromosomes differentially condensed under 5-bromodeoxyuridine treatment in cases of 49,XXXXY, 48,XXXX, 47,XXX, 46,X,i(Xq) and 45,X/46,X,i(Xq). Humangenetik 23:131-136, 1974.
46,X,i(Xq).
45,X/46,X,i(Xq).

Borgaonkar, D. S.: Unpublished data, 1974.
Patient No. 4040 in this laboratory.
Cytogenet. Cell Genet. 12:372-373, 1972.
46,X,i(Xq).
Mutant Cell Repository No. GM-88.

Caspersson, T., Lindsten, J. and Zech, L.: The nature of structural X chromosome aberrations in Turner's syndrome as revealed by quinacrine mustard fluorescence analysis. Hereditas 66:287-292, 1970.
45,X/46,X,i(Xq).
46,X,?i(Xp).

de la Chapelle, A.: Personal Communication, 1974.
45,X/46,X,dup(X).
Mutant Cell Repository No. GM-314.

de la Chapelle, A., Schroder, J. and Pernu, M.: Isochromosome for the short arm of X, a human 46,XXpi syndrome. Ann. Hum. Genet. 36:79-87, 1972.
46,X,i(Xp).
The proposita and her father were Xg(a+), and her mother was Xg(a-). These findings lend support to the suggestion that the Xg locus is on the short arm of the X chromosome.

de la Chapelle, A. and Stenstrand, K.: Dicentric human X chromosomes. Hereditas 76:259-268, 1974. Four patients with i(Xq) were studied by the Q, G and C banding techniques. Two of these abnormal X chromosomes were dicentric and the other two were monocentric. Three of these four patients were mosaics and had a 45,X cell line. A fifth patient with a large abnormal X chromosome was investigated. This chromosome was composed of two X chromosomes joined at the end of the short arms.

Dumars, K. W. and Reed, P.: Autosome-X transloc-
cation: A case report. Newport Beach, Calif.,
Birth Defects Conf., National Foundation - March
of Dimes, p. 94, June 16-21, 1974.
47,XYqs,+t(Xq;9q).

Fatora, S. R., Pan, S. F., Kenny, F. M. and
Steele, M. W.: A unique mixoploid variant of
ovarian agenesis. Amer. J. Hum. Genet. 26:30A,
1974.
46,X,i(Xq)/45,X/45,i(Xq).
This would be the first report of an Xq isochromosome persisting in a monosomic state.

Hamerton, J. L., Mohandas, T., McAlpine, P. J.
and Douglas, G. R.: Precise localization of
human gene loci using spontaneous chromosome
rearrangements in human-Chinese hamster somatic
cell hybrids. Amer. J. Hum. Genet. 26:38A, 1974.
t(X;12)(?;q21).

Kim, H. J., Hsu, L. Y. F. and Hirschhorn, K.:
Long-arm deletion with features of Turner's
syndrome. Lancet 1:1296, 1974.
46,X,i(Xq).
See also entry 0Xq200 (Wright and Scanlon, 1974).

Leisti, J. T., Kaback, M. M. and Rimoin, D. L.:
X-chromosomal and autosomal inactivation in human
X/autosomal translocations. Amer. J. Hum. Genet.
26:53A, 1974.

Sarto, G. E.: Cytogenetics of fifty patients
with primary amenorrhea. Amer. J. Obstet. Gynec.
119:14-23, 1974.
45,X/46,X,i(Xq).
46,X,i(Xq).

Solomon, I. L., Hamm, C. W. and Green, O. C.:
Chromosome studies on testicular tissue cultures
and blood leucocytes of a male previously reported to have no Y chromosome. New Eng. J. Med.
271:585-592, 1964.
46,X,i(Xq)/47,X,i(Xq),+?Y.

Stevenson, A. C., Bedford, J. and Barbertown, G.
M.: A patient with 45,X/46,XXq-/46,XXq-dic
karyotype. J. Med. Genet. 8:513-516, 1971.

45,X/46,X,Xq-/46,X,dic(X).

van den Berghe, H., Fryns, J. P. and Soyez, C.:
X/X translocation in a patient with Turner's
syndrome. Humangenetik 20:377-380, 1973.
45,X/46,X,t(X;X)(p;q).
45,X/46,X,t(X;X)(Xqter to Xp::Xq to Xqter).

van den Berghe, H., Fryns, J. P. and Devos, F.:
46,XXip karyotype in a woman with normal stature
and gonadal dysgenesis without other congenital
anomalies. Humangenetik 20:163-166, 1973.
46,X,i(Xp).
46,X,i(X)(Xpter to cen to Xpter).

Yanagisawa, S.: Isochromosome X associated with
paracentric inversion. Lancet 2:1448, 1973.
46,X/46,XX,i(Xq)/47,XX,i(Xq),i(Xq).
A paracentric inversion was hypothesized to have
occurred in the isochromosomes occurring at bands
q11 and q13 on the long arm of chromosome X.

Yanagisawa, S.: Interstitial heterochromatin in
isochromosome-X. Lancet 1:876, 1974.

Zang, K. D., Singer, H., Loeffler, L., Souvatzoglou, (NI), Halbfass, J. and Mehnert, H.: Kline-
felter-syndrom mit dem chromosomensatz 47,XXqiY.
Klin. Wschr. 47:237-244, 1969.

OXp000

Lie, G. W., Coenegracht, J. M. and Stalder, G.
R.: A very large metacentric chromosome in a
woman with symptoms of Turner's syndrome.
Cytogenetics 3:427-440, 1964.
46,X,t(X;?)(p;?).
"We conclude that the unpaired large chromosome
in our patient is an abnormal X chromosome with a
partial deletion and a translocation of a piece
of an autosome or sex chromosome onto its short
arm."

Madan, K. and Walker, S.: Possible evidence for
Xp+ in an XX male. Lancet 1:1223, 1974.
46,X,Xp+.
It is suggested that the additional material
might have come from the short arm of Y.

Neuhauser, G. and Back, F.: X-autosom-transloka-
tion bei einem kind mit multiplen Mibbildungen.
Humangenetik 3:300-311, 1967.
X-autosome translocation identified by autoradiography.

Picciano, D. J., Berlin, C. M., Lavenport, S. L.
H. and Jacobson, C. B.: Human ring chromosomes:
A report of five cases. Ann. Genet. 15:241-247,
1972.
Case No. 5 in this report.
45,X/46,X,r(X).

Ruthner, U. and Golob, E.: Fusion of the short
arms of one X chromosome in a patient with
gonadal dysgenesis. Humangenetik 24:159-160,
1974.
45,X/46,X,t(X;X)(p;p).
45,X/46,X,t(X;X)(Xqter to Xp::Xp to Xqter).

Sinha, A. K. and Nora, J. J.: Evidence for X-X
chromosome translocation in humans. Ann. Hum.
Genet. 33:117-124, 1969.
46,t(Xp+;Xq-)/45,X.
Chromosome identification by autoradiography.

van den Berghe, H.: Personal Communication,
1974.
46,X,-X,+t(Yq;Xp).

0Xp110   Negative band

Borgaonkar, D. S. and Herr, H. M.: Unpublished
observations, 1974.
Patient No. 5177 in this laboratory.
46,X,del(X)(p11q1).
46,X,del(X)(:p11 to q1:).
The minute chromosome is interpreted as a deleted
X chromosome. The patient has some features of
Turner syndrome.

Borgaonkar, D. S. and Sroka, B. M.: Unpublished
observations, 1974.
Patient No. 4989 in this laboratory.
46,X,del(X)(p11).
46,X,del(X)(qter to p11:).

Borgaonkar, D. S., Sroka, B. M. and Flores, M.:

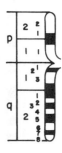

Y-to-X translocation in a girl. Lancet 1:68-69 and unpublished data, 1974.
46,X,t(X,Y)(Yqter to Yq11::Xp10 to Xq22).

Boczkowski, K. and Mikkelsen, M.: Fluorescence and autoradiographic studies in patients with Turner's syndrome and 46,XXp- and 46,XXq-karyotypes. J. Med. Genet. 10:350-355, 1973.
Case No. 1 in this report.
46,X,del(X)(p11).
46,X,del(X)(qter to p11:).

Buckton, K. E., Jacobs, P. A., Rae, L. A., Newton, M. S. and Sanger, R.: An inherited X-autosome translocation in man. Ann. Hum. Genet. 35:171-178, 1971.
45,X/46,XX,p-.
46,X and Y,t(X;14)(p11;q32).
46,X,der(X)der(14)t(X;14)(p11;q32)mat.
Chromosome identification by autoradiography.
See report by Jacobs et al. (1974).

Chrz, R., Kozak, J. and Malkova, J.: Densitometric study of G bands on human metaphase chromosomes. Humangenetik 18:149-154, 1973.
del(X)(p1).
del(X)(qter to p1:).

Fellous, M: Rotterdam Conference, 1974.
t(X;17)(p11;q20).

Jacobs, P. A., Buckton, K. E., Cunningham, C. and Newton, M. S.: An analysis of the break points of structural rearrangements in man. J. Med. Genet. 11:50-64, 1974.
M. R. C. Registry No. K24-60-66 in this report.
46,X,t(X;14)(p11;q32).
See report by Buckton et al. (1974).

Pearson, P. L., van der Linden, A. G. J. M. and Hagemeijer, A.: Localization of gene markers to regions of the human X chromosome by segregation of X-autosome translocations in somatic cell hybrids. Birth Defects: Original Article Series X(3):136-142, 1974. Cited by Gerald, P. S. and Brown, J. A.:29-34.
t(X;17)(p11;p13).

van den Berghe, H.: Personal Communication,
1974.
46,X,del(X)(p11).
46,X,der del(X)(p11).
46,X,der del(X)(Xqter to Xp11:).
No stigmata of Turner syndrome or gonadal dysgenesis.

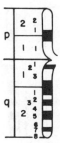

OXp114   Negative band

Styles, S. M.: Evidence on the origin of an
apparent X isochromosome in man: Trypsin-Giemsa
banding. Twelfth Ann. Somatic Cell Genet. Conf.,
Utah, 80, 1974.
46,X,-X+t(X;X)(p114,q13).
46,X,-X,+t(X;X)(Xqter to cen to p114::q13 to
qter).

OXp120   Positive band

Pearson, P. L., van der Linden, A. G. J. M. and
Hagemeijer, A.: Localization of gene markers to
regions of the human X chromosome by segregation
of X-autosome translocations in somatic cell
hybrids. Birth Defects: Original Article Series
X(3):136-142, 1974. Cited by Gerald, P. S. and
Brown, J. A.:29-34.
t(X;8)(p12;p22).

OXp200

Khudr, G. and Benirschke, K.: X/Y translocation.
Amer. J. Obstet. Gynec. 116:584-585, 1973.
46,X,t(X,Y)(p2;q1).
46,X,t(X,Y)(Xqter to Xp2::4q1 to Yqter).
See Khudr et al. (1973) in entry OXp220.

Mukerjee, D. and Burdette, W. J.: Multiple
congenital anomalies associated with a ring 3
chromosome and translocated 3/X chromosome.
Nature 212:135-155, 1966.
46,r(3)(pq),t(X;3)(p2;p or q).
46,r(3)(p to q),t(X;3)(Xqter to Xp2::3p or q to
3pter or 3qter).

Thelen, T. H., Abrams, D. J. and Fisch, R. O.:
Multiple abnormalities due to possible genetic
inactivation in an X/autosome translocation.

Amer. J. Hum. Genet. 23:410-418, 1971.
46,X,t(X;18)(p2;q1).

OXp210   Positive band

Hamerton, J. L., Mohandas, T., McAlpine, P. J.
and Douglas, G. R.: Precise localization of
human gene loci using spontaneous chromosome
rearrangements in human-Chinese hamster somatic
cell hybrids. Amer. J. Hum. Genet. 26:38A, 1974.

OXp220   Negative band

Disteche, C., Hagemeijer, A., Frederic, J. and
Progneaux, D.: An abnormal large human chromosome identified as an end-to-end fusion of two
X's by combined results of the new banding
techniques and microdensitometry. Clin. Genet.
3:388-395, 1972.
46,X,-X,+t(X;X)(p22;p22).
46,X,-X,+t(X;X)(Xqter to Xp22::Xp22 to Xqter).
The centromeric region of one of the translocated
X chromosomes does not function as a centromere,
i.e., the translocated chromosome is not dicentric.

Khudr, G., Benirschke, K., Judd, H. L. and
Strauss, J.:   Y to X translocation in a woman
with reproductive failure.   JAMA 226:544-549,
1973.
46,X,t(X;Y)(p22;q11).
46,X,t(X;Y)(Xqter to Xp22::Yq11 to Yqter).
See Khudr and Benirschke (1973) in entry OXp200.

Mikkelsen, M. and Dahl, G.: Unbalanced X-autosomal translocation with inactivation of the
normal X chromosome.   Cytogenet. Cell Genet.
12:357-366, 1973.
46,X,t(X;8)(p22;q21).
46,X,t(X;8)(Xqter to p22::8q21 to 8qter).

Wie Lie, G., Coenegracht, J. M. and Stalder, G.
R.:   A very large metacentric chromosome in a
woman with symptoms of Turner's syndrome.
Cytogenetics 3:427-430, 1964.

OXq000

Allderdice, P. W., Miller, O. J., Klinger, H. P.,
Pallister, P. D. and Opitz, J. M.: Demonstration
of a spreading effect in an X-autosome translocation by combined autoradiographic and quinacrine-
fluorescence studies. Excerpta Medica, Fourth
Int. Cong. Hum. Genet. 233:14, 1971.
46,X,t(Xq-;14q+).
47,Y,-X,-14,-14,+der(X)+der(14)+der(14)t(Xq-;14q+
)mat.
See Opitz, Pallister and Ruddle (1973) in entry
0Xq130.

Same entry as in 09q000 (Dumars, Reed and Lawce,
1974).

Lubs, H. A.: A marker X chromosome. Amer. J.
Hum. Genet. 21:231-244, 1969.
A secondary constriction near the end of the long
arm giving the appearance of large satellites was
found in males and females in a kindred.

Mann, J. D. and Higgins, J.: A case of primary
amenorrhea associated with X-autosomal translocation [46,X,t(Xq-;5q+)]. Amer. J. Hum. Genet.
26:416, 1974.
46,X,t(Xq-;5q+).

Sarto, G. E.: Cytogenetics of fifty patients
with primary amenorrhea. Amer. J. Obstet. Gynec.
119:14-23, 1974.
46,X,t(Xq-;12q+).

Therman, E., Sarto, G. E. and Patau, K.: Center
for Barr body condensation on the proximal part
of the human Xq: A hypothesis. Chromosoma
44:361-366, 1974.

Same entry as in 0X0000 (van den Berghe, Fryns
and Soyez, 1973).

0Xq100

Bocian, M., Krompotic, E., Szego, K. and Rosenthal, I. M.: Somatic stigmata of Turner's
syndrome in a patient with 46,XXq-. J. Med.
Genet. 8:358-363, 1971.
46,X,del(X)(q1).
46,X,del(X)(pter to q1:).

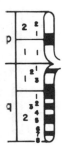

Same entry as in 0Xp110 (Borgaonkar and Herr, 1974).

Cohen, M. M., Lin, C. C., Sybert, V. and Orecchio, E. J.: Two human X-autosome translocations identified by autoradiography and fluorescence. Amer. J. Hum. Genet. 24:583-597, 1972.
Patient No. 1 in this report.
46,X,t(X;9)(q1;p2).

Luthardt, F. W. and Palmer, C. G.: X chromosome long arm deletion in a patient with Down's syndrome. J. Med. Genet. 8:387-391, 1971.
47,X,del(X)(q1),+21.
47,X,del(X)(pter to q1:),+21.

0Xq110   Negative band

Leisti, J.: The Turner phenotype associated with unbalanced X/autosome translocation. Newport Beach, Calif., Birth Defects Conf., National Foundation - March of Dimes, pp. 193-194, June 16-21, 1974.
46,X,t(X;9)(q11;q32).
Case MH 620082 in this report.
46,X,-X,+der(9)t(X;9)(q11;q32)mat.
46,X,-X,+der(9)t(X;9)(9pter to 9q32::Xq11 to Xqter)mat.

Summitt, R. L., Martens, P. R. and Wilroy, R. S.: X-autosome translocation in normal mother and effectively 21-monosomic daughter. J. Pediat. 84:539-546, 1974.
46,X,t(X;21)(q11;p11?).
46,X,t(X;21)(Xpter to Xq11::21p11? to 21pter;21qter to 21p11?::Xq11 to Xqter).
46,XX,-21,+der(21),t(X;21)(q11;p11?)mat.
46,XX,-21,+der(21),t(X;21)(21qter to 21p11?::Xq11 to Xqter)mat.
A good summary of 20 previously reported X-autosome translocations can be found in tiis report.

Same entry as in 0X0000 (Yanagisawa, 1973).

0Xq112   Negative band

Ruthner, U. and Golob, E.: Identification of a

large submetacentric X chromosome as pericentric
inversion of an isochromosome cf the long arm.
Humangenetik 22:171-175, 1974.
46,X,inv[i(Xq)](q113q112) or
46,X,inv[i(Xq)](1stXqter to 1stXq13::2ndXq12 to
1stXq13::2ndXq12 to 2ndXqter).
The isochromosome consists of two long arms.
They are identified as 1stXq and 2ndXq.

OXq120   Positive band

Shows, T. B. and Brown, J. A.: An (Xq+;9p-)
translocation suggests the assignment of G6PD,
HPRT, and PGK to the long arm of the X chromosome
in somatic cell hybrids. Birth Defects: Original
Article Series X(3):146-149, 1974.
46,X,t(X,9)(q12;p24).
46,X,t(X,9)(Xpter to Xq12;9qter to 9p24::Xq12 to
Xqter).
Normal X chromosome is inactive.

OXq130   Negative band

Lucas, M. and Smithies, A.: Banding patterns and
autoradiographic studies of cells with an X-
autosome translocation. Ann. Hum. Genet. 37:9-
12, 1974.
46,X,t(X;15)(q13;p13).

Opitz, J. M., Pallister, D. and Ruddle, F. H.:
An (X;14) translocation, balanced, 46 chromosomes. Cytogenet. Cell Genet. 12:289-290, 1973.
46,X,t(X;14)(q13;q32).
46,X,t(X;14)(Xpter to Xq13::?14q32 to 14qter;14p-
ter to 14q32::Xq13 to Xqter).
Mutant Cell Repository No. GM-73, KOP-1.

Opitz, J. M., Pallister, D. and Ruddle, F. H.:
An (X;14) translocation, unbalanced, 47 chromosomes. Cytogenet. Cell Genet. 12:290-291, 1973.
47,Y,-X,-14,+der(X)+der(14)+
der(14)t(X;14)(q13;q32)mat.
Mutant Cell Repository No. GM-74,KOP-2.

Rary, J. M.: Personal Communication, 1974).
Case No. 1008 in this laboratory.
46,X,del(X)(q13).
46,X,del(X)(pter to q13:).

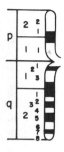

Ricciuti, F. C. and Ruddle, F. H.: Assignment of three gene loci (PGK, HGPRT, G6PD) to the long arm of the human X chromosome by somatic cell genetics. Genetics 74:661-678, 1973.
See Opitz, Pallister and Ruddle (1973) in entry 0Xq130.

Same entry as in 0Xq112 (Ruthner and Golob, 1974).

Stoll, C., Muller, P. and Dellenbach, P.: X deletion and primary amenorrhoea. Lancet 1:436, 1973.
46,X,del(X)(q13).
46,X,del(X)(pter to q13:).

Same entry as in 0Xp114 (Styles, 1974).

Same entry as in 0X0000 (Yanagisawa, 1973).

0Xq200

Chandra, H. S., Reddy, G. N., Peter, J. and Venkatachalaiah, G.: A 47,XXq-Y Klinefelter male. J. Med. Genet. 8:530-532, 1971.
47,XY,del(X)(q2).
47,XY,del(X)(pter to q2:).

Cohen, M. M., Lin, C. C., Sybert, V. and Orecchio, E. J.: Two human X-autosome translocations identified by autoradiography and fluorescence. Amer. J. Hum. Genet. 24:583-597, 1972.
Patient No. 2 in this report.
46,X,t(X;8)(q2;q1).

Dutrillaux, B.: Chromosomal aspects of human male sterility. Nobel Symposium 23:205-208, 1972.
46,X,t(X;1)(q2;q2).
46,Y,der(X)der(1)t(X;1)(q2;q2)mat.

Gerald, P. S.: Personal Communication, 1974.
46,X,t(X;19)(q22 to 24;q13 or p13).
Mutant Cell Repository No. GM-89.
Normal X chromosome is inactive.

Hecht, F., Jones, D. L., Delay, M. and Klevit, H.: Xq- Turner's syndrome: reconsideration of

hypothesis that Xp- causes somatic features in Turner's syndrome. J. Med. Genet. 7:1-4, 1970.
46,X,del(X)(q2).
46,X,del(X)(pter to q2:).

Jacobs, P. A., Buckton, K. E., Cunningham, C. and Newton, M. S.: An analysis of the break points in structural rearrangements in man. J. Med. Genet. 11:50-64, 1974.
M. R. C. Repository No. K111-47-69 in this report.
46,X,t(X;2)(q2;q2).

Sarto, G. E., Therman, E. and Patau, K.: X-inactivation in man: A woman with t(Xq-;12q+). Amer. J. Hum. Genet. 25:262-270, 1973.
46,X,t(X;12)(q2;q2).
46,X,t(X;12)(Xpter to Xq2::12q2 to 12qter;12pter to 12q2::Xq2 to Xqter).

Therman, E., Sarto, G. E., and Patau, K.: Apparently isodicentric but functionally monocentric X chromosome in man. Amer. J. Hum. Genet. 26:83-92, 1974.
46,X,-X,+dic(X)(q2).
46,X,-X,+dic(X)(Xpter to Xq2::Xq2 to Xpter).
Also contains a fine table, which lists previously reported unbalanced X translocation cases.

Wright, E. V. and Scanlon, M. F.: X long-arm deletion with features of Turner's syndrome. Lancet 1:933, 1974.
46,X,del(X)(q2).
46,X,del(X)(pter to q2:).

0Xq210   Positive band

Boczkowski, K. and Mikkelsen, M.: Fluorescence and autoradiographic studies in patients with Turner's syndrome and 46,XXp- and 46,XXq- karyotypes. J. Med. Genet. 10:350-355, 1973.
Case No. 2 in this report.
46,X,del(X)(q21).
46,X,del(X)(pter to q21:).

0Xq220   Negative band

Same entry as in 0Xp100 (Borgaonkar, Sroka and

Flores, 1974).

Brown, J. A., Shows, T. B. and Palmer, C. G.:
Rotterdam Conference, 1974.
46,X,t(X;22)(q22;q13).

0Xq230   Positive band

Pearson, P. L., van der Linden, A. G. J. M. and
Hagemeijer, A.: Localization of gene markers to
regions of the human X chromosome by segregation
of X-autosome translocations in somatic cell
hybrids. Birth Defects: Original Article Series
X(3):136-142, 1974. Cited by Gerald, P. S. and
Brown, J. A.:29-34.
t(X;22)(q23;q13).

0Xq240   Negative band

Same entry as in 0Xp210 (Hamerton et al., 1974).

Rary, J. M.: Personal Communication, 1974.
Case No. 195 in this laboratory.
45,X/46,X,del(X)(q24).
45,X/46,X,del(X)(pter to q24:).

0Xq260   Negative band

Pearson, P. L., van der Linden, A. G. J. M. and
Hagemeijer, A.: Localization of gene markers to
regions of the human X chromosome by segregation
of X-autosome translocations in somatic cell
hybrids. Birth Defects: Original Article Series
X(3):136-142, 1974. Cited by Gerald, P. S. and
Brown, J. A.:29-34.
t(X;3)(q26;q12).
See entry 0Xq280 (de la Chapelle and Schroder,
1974). Pearson et al. acknowledge receiving
translocation material from Dr. de la Chapelle
and may be in fact reporting on the same cell
line.

Punnett, H. H., Kistenmacher, M. L., Greene, A.
E. and Coriell, L. L.: An (X;1) translocation,
balanced, 46 chromosomes. Repository identification No. GM-97. Cytogenet. Cell Genet. 13:406-
407, 1974.
46,X,t(X;1)(q26;q12).

46,X,t(X;1)(Xpter to Xq26::1q12 to 1qter;1pter to 1q12::Xq26 to Xqter).
Mutant Cell Repository No. GM-97.

Sanger, R., Alfi, O. S. and Donnell, G. N.: Partial trisomy 1q in 3 patients. Amer. J. Hum. Genet. 26:75A, 1974.
46,X,-X,+t(X;1)(q26;q32).
46,X,-X,+t(X;1)(Xpter to Xq26::1q32 to 1qter).

0Xq270   Positive band

Crandall, B. F., Carrel, R. E., Howard, J., Schroeder, W. A. and Muller, H.: Trisomy 13 with a 13-X translocation. Amer. J. Hum. Genet. 26:385-392, 1974.
46,X,-X,+t(X;13)(q27;q12).
46,X,-X,+t(X;13)(Xpter to Xq27::13q12 to 13qter).
A 15 month old girl with some features of trisomy 13 is described.
The patient is monosomic for Xq27 and Xq28 band regions of X chromosome, and partially trisomic for chromosome 13q12 to q terminal region.

0Xq280   Negative band

de la Chapelle, A. and Schroder, J.: Apparently non-reciprocal balanced human (3q-;Xq+) translocation: Late replication of structurally normal X. Chromosomes Today 4:261-265, 1974.
46,X,t(X;3)(q28;q13).
46,X,t(X;3)(Xpter to Xq28::3q13 to 3qter;3pter to 3q13::?).
The normal X chromosome is inactive.
See entry 0Xq230 (Pearson et al., 1974). It may be that the cell line that they report on is the same that is reported here. If so, there is obviously an error in determining the exact break point since they report it at Xq26 and 3q12.

Engel, W., Vogel, W. and Reinwein, H.: Autoradiographic studies on an X-autosomal translocation in man: 45,X,15-,tan(15qXq+)+. Cytogenetics 10:87-98, 1971.
45,X,-15,+tan(X;15)(q28;q1).
45,X,-15,+tan(X;15)(Xpter to Xq28::15q1 to 15qter).
Chromosome identification by autoradiography.

Klinger, H. P. and de la Chapelle, A.: Personal Communication, 1974.
46,X,t(X;3)(q28;q13).
Mutant Cell Repository No. GM-194.

p | | |
q | | 2   0Y0000

Armendares, S., Buentello, L., Salamanca, F. and Cantu-Garza, J. M.: A dicentric Y chromosome without evidence of sex chromosomal mosaicism, 46,XYqdic, in a patient with features of Turner's syndrome. J. Med. Genet. 9:96-100, 1972.
46,X,dic(Y).

Berger, R., Lejeune, J. and Roy, J.: Trisomie 21 et Y metacentrique. Ann. Genet. 13:187-197, 1973.
46,X,Yq-.
46,X,der(Yq-)pat.
47,X,der(Yq-)pat,+21.

Book, J. A., Eilon, B., Halbrecht, I., Komlos, L. and Shabtay, F.: Isochromosome Y [46,X,i(Yq)] and female phenotype. Clin. Genet. 4:410-414, 1973.
46,X,i(Yq).

Jacobs, P. A. and Ross, A.: Structural abnormalities of the Y chromosome in man. Nature 210:352-354, 1966.
Cases 1 and 2 in this report.
46,X,i(Yq).

Jones, K. W.: Rotterdam Conference, 1974.
t(Y;13).

Meisner, L. F. and Inhorn, S. L.: Normal male development with Y chromosome long arm deletion (Yq-). J. Med. Genet. 19:373-377, 1972.
46,X,del(Y)(q11:) or 46,X,i(Yp).

Nakagome, Y., Smith, H. D. and Soukup, S. W.: A presumptive Y-autosome translocation in a boy with congenital malformations. Amer. J. Dis. Child. 116:205-210, 1968.
47,XY,+t(Yq?Gq).

Park, I. J., Heller, R. H., Jones, H. W. and

Woodruff, J. D.: Apparent pseudopuberty in a
phenotypic female with a gonadal tumor and an
autosome/Y chromosome translocation. Amer. J.
Obstet. Gynec. 119:661-668, 1974.
45,X,-16,+t(Yq16q)/46,XYq,-16,+t(Yq16q).

Ruthner, U. and Golob, E.: 45,Y/45,X,ace(?Yp)+/
46,X,r(Y) in a phenotypically normal newborn
male. Humangenetik 22:177-180, 1974.

Siebers, J. W., Vogel, W., Hepp, H., Bolze, H.
and Dittrich, A.: Structural aberrations of the
Y chromosome and the corresponding phenotype.
Report of a case with the karyotype 45,X/
46,X,i(Yp). Humangenetik 19:57-66, 1973.
45,X/46,X,i(Yp).
A good review on the localization of sex-determining factors on the Y chromosone.

Sulica, L. O., Borgaonkar, D. S. and Shah, S. A.:
Accurate identification of the human Y chromosome. Clin. Genet. 5:17-27, 1974.

van den Berghe, H.: Personal Communication,
1974.
A Y/Y translocation in a newborn male with
craniosynostosis.

van den Berghe, H., Steeno, O., Verresen, H. and
de Moor, P.: Hypogonadism associated with
chromosomal break in autosome No. 2 and translocation presumably on the Y chromosome. J. Clin.
Endocr. 25:1246-1250, 1965.
See entry OYp110 (van den Berghe, Fryns and
David, 1973).

OYp110   Negative band

Baheux, G., Emerit, I. and Roux, C.: Trisomie 21
et anomalie de structure de L'Y. Ann. Genet.
13:191-194, 1970.
46,X,inv(Y)(pq).
47,X,inv(Y)(pq),+21.

Bochkov, N. P., Kuleshov, N. P., Chebotarev, A.
N., Alekhin, V. I. and Midian, S. A.: Population
cytogenetic investigation of newborns in Moscow.
Humangenetik 22:139-152, 1974.

46,X,inv(Y)(p+q-)pat.

Borgaonkar, D. S.: Application of new technics of chromosome identification to cytogenetic problems. Birth Defects: Original Article Series Vol. IX, No. 1:171-182, 1973.
A case of pericentric Y inversion is described.
46,XY,inv(Y)(p11q1).
46,XY,inv(Y)(pter to p11::q1 to p11::q1 to qter).

Buhler, E. M., Frey, R., Muller, H., Voegdin, M. and Stalder, G. R.: Fluorescence pattern of a dicentric Y. Humangenetik 12:170-172, 1971.
46,XY,dic(Y).

Chandley, A. C. and Edmond, P.: Meiotic studies on a subfertile patient with a ring Y chromosome. Cytogenetics 10:295-304, 1971.
45,X/46,X,r(Y).
Purportedly first report of a ring Y chromosome in man. The X and the ring Y remained unpaired at diakinesis and maturation arrest between the first and second meiotic divisions was observed.

Cohen, M. M., MacGillivray, M. H., Capraro, V. J. and Aceto, T. A.: Human dicentric Y chromosomes: case report and review of the literature. J. Med. Genet. 10:74-79, 1973.
45,X/46,X,dic(Yq).

Czeizel, A., Csosz, L., Gardonyi, J., Remenar, L. and Ruzicska, P.: Chromosome studies in twelve patients with retinoblastoma. Humangenetik 22:159-166, 1974.
46,X,inv(Y)(pq).

de Almeida, J. C. C., Barcinski, M. A., doceu Abreu, M., Naya, J., Kayath, H. C., Cunha, A. G., Schulz, I., Mello, R. S. and Santos, R. R.: 45,X/46,XY,r(Y) in a case of asymmetrical testicular differentiation. Ann. Genet. 17:37-40, 1974.
45,X/46,X,r(Y).
Since the patient presented with asymmetrical testicular differentiation, the possibility that the male determining factors must be located on either arms of the Y chromosome near the centromere is discussed.

Friedrich, U. and Nielsen, J.: Pericentric inversion Y in a population of newborn boys. Hereditas 76:147-152, 1974.
Proband Nos. 7890 and 9748 in this report.
46,X,inv(Y)(p11q11).
46,X,inv(Y)(pter to p11::q11 to p11::q11 to qter).

German, J., Simpson, J. L. and McLemore, G. A.: Abnormalities of human sex chromcsomes. I. A ring Y without mosaicism. Ann. Genet. 16:225-231, 1973.
46,X,r(Y)(pq).

Grace, H. J., Ally, F. E. and Paruk, M. A.: 46,X,inv(Yp+q-) in four generations of an Indian family. J. Med. Genet. 9:293-297, 1972.
46,X,inv(Y)(pq).
46,X,der(Y)inv(Y)(pq)pat.

Jacobs, P. A., Price, W. H., Richmond, S. and Ratcliff, R. A. W.: Chromosome surveys in penal institutions and approved schools. J. Med. Genet. 8:49-58, 1971.
Cases 211-68 and 245-68 in this report.
46,X,inv(Y)(pq).

Jacobs, P. A. and Ross, A.: Structural abnormalities of the Y chromosome in man. Nature 210:352-354, 1966.
Case No. 3 in this report.
46,X,inv(Y)(pq).
Case No. 4 in this report.
46,XX,inv(Y)(pq).

Krompotic, E., Szego, K., Modestas, R. and Molabola, G. B.: Localization of male determining factor on short arm of Y chromosome. Case report of a baby with 46,X,t(Yp+;14q-). Clin. Genet. 3:381-387, 1972.
46,X,t(Y;14)(p11;q2).
Mutant Cell Repository No. GM-28⊾.

Khudr, G. and Benirschke, K.: Y ring chromosome associated with gonadoblastoma in situ. Obstet. Gynec. 41:897-901, 1973.
45,X/46,X,r(Y).

Lauritsen, J. G., Jonasson, J., Therkelsen, A. J., Lass, F., Lindsten, J. and Petersen, G. B.: Studies on spontaneous abortions. Fluorescence analysis of abnormal karyotypes. Hereditas 71:160-163, 1972.
48,inv(Y)(pq),+16,+18.

Sarto, G. E., Opitz, J. M. and Inhorn, S. L.: Considerations of sex chromosome abnormalities in man. In Comparative Mammalian Cytogenetics, Benirschke, K. Ed. Springer-Verlag, New York:390-413, 1969.
Case 1 D.Z. 011250 in this report.
46,XX/47,XX,r(Y).

Sparkes, R. S., Muller, H. M. and Veomett, I. C.: Inherited pericentric inversion of a human Y chromosome in trisomic Down's syndrome. J. Med. Genet. 7:59-62, 1970.
46,X,inv(Y)(pq).
46,X,der(Y)inv(Y)(pq)pat.
47,X,der(Y)inv(Y)(pq)pat,+21.

Subrt, I. and Blehova, B.: Robertsonian translocation between the chromosome Y and 15. Humangenetik 23:305-309, 1974.
45,X,-Y,-15,+t(Y;15)(p11;q11).
45,X,-Y,-15,+t(Y;15)(Yqter to Yp11::15q11 to 15qter).

van den Berghe, H., Fryns, J. P. and David, G.: An autosome-Y translocation restudied. Humangenetik 20:375-376, 1973.
46,X,t(2;Y)(p1;p11).

Ying, K. L. and Ives, E. J.: Mitotic behavior of human dicentric Y chromosomes. Cytogenetics 10:208-218, 1971.
45,X/46,X,dic(Y)(p11).

Zeuthen, E. and Nielsen, J.: Pericentric Y inversion in the general population. Humangenetik 19:265-270, 1973.
There are no indications that pericentric Y inversion is associated with phenotypic deviation.

0Yq100

Borgaonkar, D. S., McKusick, V. A., Herr, H. M., de los Cobos, L. and Yoder, O. C.: Constancy of the length of human Y chromosome. Ann. Genet. 12:262-264, 1969.
46,X,Yq+ and 46,X,Yq-.
Family studies showing variations in the length of the Y chromosome have been reported.

Caspersson, T., Hulten, M., Jonasson, J., Lindsten, J., Therkelsen, A. J. and Zech, L.: Translocations causing non-fluorescent Y chromosomes in human XO/XY mosaics. Hereditas 68:317-324, 1971.
Case No. 4 in this report.
45,X/46,X,t(Y;2)(q1;p).
A patient with a nonfluorescent Y chromosome is hypothesized to have a t(2p+;Yc-) translocation on the basis of results obtained with meiotic material.

Same entry as in 09q000 (Dumars, Reed and Lawce, 1974).

Friedrich, U. and Nielsen, J.: Presumptive Y-15 and Y-22 translocations in two families. Hereditas 71:339-342, 1972.
Case report A.
46,XX,-15,+t(Y;15)(q1;p1).
46,XX,-15,+t(Y;15)(15qter to 15p1::Yq1 to Yqter).
46,XY,-15,+der(15)t(Y;15)(q1;p1)mat.
Proband No. 173 in this report.
46,XY,-15,+der(15)t(Y;15)(q1;p1)mat.
Case report B.
46,XX,-22,+t(Y;22)(q1;p1).
46,XX,-22,+t(Y;22)(22qter to 22p1::Yq1 to Yqter).
46,XY,-22,+der(22)t(Y;22)(q1;p1)mat.
Proband No. 27 in this report.
46,XX,-22,+der(22)t(Y;22)(q1;p1)mat.

Frund, S., Koske-Westphal, T., Fuchs-Mecke, S. and Passarge, E.: Quinacrine mustard fluorescence of a second Y chromosome in a Y-autosomal translocation. Humangenetik 14:133-136, 1972.
Translocation of the fluorescent segment of the Y to the short arm of 15 has been hypothesized:
46,XY,t(Y;15)(q1;p1).

Genest, P.: Hereditary transmission since 300

years of a satellited Y chromosome in a family.
Ann. Genet. 16:35-38, 1973.

Genest, P.: A human satellited Y chromosome with
a probably illegitimate paternal origin. Canad.
Med. Ass. J. 107:1205-1206, 1972.
Family A in this report.
46,X,Yqs.
46,X,der(Yqs)pat.

Genest, P., Bouchard, M. and Bouchard, J.: A
satellited human Y chromosome: an evidence of
autosome gonosome translocation. A preliminary
note. Canad. J. Genet. Cytol. 9:589-595, 1967.
46,X,Yqs.
46,X,der(Yqs)pat.
47,X,der(Yqs)pat,+21.

Genest, P. and Lejeune, J.: On the origin of a
small Y chromosome several hundred years old.
Ann. Genet. 15:51-53, 1972.

Gilgenkrantz, S., Pierson, M. and Mauuary, G.:
13q+ chromosome due to a probable translocation
of a supernumerary Y. Ann. Genet. 16:167-172,
1973.
46,XY,t(Y;13)(q1;q).
46,XY,t(Y;13)(13pter to 13q::Yq1 to Yqter).

Same entry as in 15p100 (Hahnemann and Eiberg,
1973).

Kyaosaar, M. E. and Mikelsaar, A. V. N.: Chromosome investigation in married couples with
repeated abortions. Humangenetik 17:277-283,
1973.
Case Nos. 7 and 16 in this report.
46,X,Yq+.

Same entry as in 0Xp200 (Khudr and Benirschke,
1973).

Leisti, J.: Structural variation in human
mitotic chromosomes. Ann. Acad. Sci. fenn.
(Med.) Series A, IV, Biologica 179:1-69, 1971.
Case No. 20 in this report.
47,X,t(Yq;?6q),+21.

McKenzie, W. H., Hostetter, T. L. and Lubs, H. A.: Y family study: Heritable variation in the length of the human Y chromosome. Amer. J. Hum. Genet. 24:686-693, 1971.

Miller, R. C., Goodman, R. M., Miller, F. R. and Nusbaum, L.: A new variant of Klinefelter's syndrome with a presumptive deleted Y chromosome. Ann. Intern. Med. 67:825-831, 1967.
46,XX,del(Y)(q1).
46,XX,del(Y)(pter to q1:).

Same entry as in 05p150 (Nakagome, Iinuma and Taniguchi, 1973).

Nielsen, J., Friedrich, U. and Tsuboi, T.: Father and son with karyotype 47,XY,?Yq-. Humangenetik 11:247-252, 1971.
47,XY,+Yq-.
47,XY,+der(Yq-)pat.

Reitalu, J.: A familial Y-22 translocation in man. Hereditas 74:155-160, 1973.
46,XX,-22,+t(Y;22)(q1;p1).
46,XX,-22,+t(Y;22)(22qter to 22p1::Yq1 to Yqter).
46,XY,-22,+der(22)t(Y;22)(q1;p1)mat.

Ruzicska, P. and Czeizel, A.: Cytogenetic studies on mid-trimester abortuses. Humangenetik 10:273-297, 1970.
Abortus No. 70-67 in this report.
46,XY,Yq+,16q+.

Soudek, D., Langmuir, V. and Stewart, O. J.: Variation in the nonfluorescent segment of long Y chromosome. Humangenetik 18:285-290, 1973.

Sperling, K. and Lackman, I.: Large human Y chromosome with two fluorescent bands. Clin. Genet. 2:352-355, 1971.
46,X,dup(Y)(q1).

Same entry as in 0Xp000 (van den Berghe, 1974).

0Yq110   Negative band

Bengtsson, B., Gustavson, K. E., Reuterskiold, G., Santesson, B. and Ahnsen, S.: Male pseudo-

hermaphroditism with a 45X/46,XYq-/mosaicism in a pair of monozygotic twins. Clin. Genet. 5:133-143, 1974.
45,X/46,X,del(Y)(q11).
45,X/46,X,del(Y)(pter to q11:).

Same entry as in 0Xp100 (Borgaonkar, Sroka and Flores, 1974).

Develing, A. J., Conte, F. A. and Epstein, C. J.: A Y-autosome translocation 46,X,t(Yq-:7q+) associated with multiple congenital anomalies. J. Pediat. 82:495-498, 1973.
46,X,t(Y;7)(q11;q3).

Same entry as in 0Yp110 (Friedrich and Nielsen, 1974).

Same entry as in 0Xp220 (Khudr et al., 1973).

Nielsen, J. and Friedrich, U.: A phenotypic male with karyotype 45,X/45,X,ace+(?yq-). Humangenetik 15:319-329, 1972.
45,X/45,X,del(Y)(q11).
45,X/45,X,del(Y)(pter to q11:).

Pfeiffer, R. A., Bier, L., Majeinski, F. and Rager, K.: De novo translocation t(Yq-;15p+) in a malformed boy. Humangenetik 19:349-352, 1973. Patient No. WS 651004 in this report.
46,X,t(Y;15)(q11;p1).

Warburton, D. and Bluming, A.: "Philadelphia-like" chromosome derived from the Y in a patient with refractory dysplastic anemia. Blood 42:799-804, 1973.
46,X,del(Y)(q11).
46,X,del(Y)(pter to q11:).

Ying, K. L. and Ives, E. J.: Human dicentric Y chromosomes. Amer. J. Hum. Genet. 26:96A, 1974.
45,X/46,X,dic(Y)(q11).

0Yq120   Variable band

Borgaonkar, D. S. and Hollander, D. H.: Quinacrine fluorescence of the human Y chromosome. Nature 230:52, 1971.

46,XY,del(Y)(q12).
46,XY,del(Y)(pter to q12:).
46,XY,dic(Y).

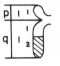

It was first pointed out here that the bright fluorescent segment of the long arm is not necessary for maleness.

Knuutila, S. and Gripenberg, U.: The fluorescence pattern of a human Yq+ chromosome. Hereditas 70:307-308, 1972.

Reitalu, J., Bergman, S., Ekwall, B. and Hall, B.: Correlation between Y chromosome length and fluorescence intensity of Y chromatin on interphase nuclei. Hereditas 72:261-268, 1972.

Zech, L.: Investigation of metaphase chromosomes with DNA-binding fluorochromes. Exp. Cell Res. 58:463, 1969.
The characteristic brightly fluorescent segment of the long arm of the human Y chromosome was first reported here.

0Yq121   Variable band

Same entry as in 21p120 (Hillman et al., 1974).

0Yq122   Negative band

Lundsten, C. and Philip, J.: Y/22 translocation in a YY male. Cytogenet. Cell Genet. 12:53-59, 1973.
46,XY,-22,+t(Y;22)(q122;p12).
46,XY,-22,+t(Y;22)(22qter to 22p12::Yq122 to Yqter).

For lack of any other suitable place the following entries are placed here.

XX MALE

Anderson, L., Bergman, S., Reitalu, J. and Anselm, S.: A case of XX male. Cytogenetic findings by autoradiography and fluorescence. Hereditas 70:311-314, 1972.

de la Chapelle, A.: Nature and origin of males with XX sex chromosomes. Amer. J. Hum. Genet. 24:71-105, 1972.

Kasdan, R., Nankin, H. R., Troen, P., Wald, N., Pan, S. F. and Yanaihara, T.: Paternal transmission of maleness in XX human beings. New Eng. J. Med. 288:539-545, 1973.

Same entry as in 0Xp000 (Madan and Walker, 1974).

Nicolis, G. L., Hsu, L. Y. F., Sabetghadam, R., Kardon, N. B., Chernay, P. R., Mathur, D. P., Rose, H. G., Hirschhorn, K. and Gabrilove, J. L.: Klinefelter's syndrome in identical twins with the 46,XX chromosome constitution. Amer. J. Med. 52:482-491, 1972.

Same entry as in 0X+ - 47,XXY (Palutke, Chen and Chen, 1973).

46,XY FEMALE (Gonadal dysgenesis).

Hill, J. A. and McKenna, H.: Pure gonadal dysgenesis. An XY female with gonadoblastoma and adenofibroma. Aust. N.Z. J. Obstet Gynaec. 14:50-52, 1974.

46,XY FEMALE (Gonadal agenesis).

Sarto, G. E. and Opitz, J. M.: The XY gonadal agenesis syndrome. J. Med. Genet. 10:288-293, 1973.

XX - XY CHIMERA

Benirschke, K.: Chimerism, mosaicism and hy-
brids. In Human Genetics, Proc. Fourth Int'l.
Conq. Hum. Genet. de Grouchy, J., Ebbing, F. J.
G. and Henderson, I. W., Editors. Excerpta
Medica, Amsterdam:212-231, 1972.
46,XX/46,XY chimera.

Corey, M. J., Miller, J. R., MacLean, J. R. and
Chown, B.: A case of XX/XY mosaicism. Amer. J.
Hum. Genet. 19:378-387, 1967.
It is concluded on the basis of studies on blood
groups, karyotype and phenotype that the boy is a
product of fertilization of two female elements
by two sperm.

Park, I. J., Jones, H. W. and Bias, W. B.: True
hermaphroditism with 46,XX/46,XY chromosome
complement. Report of a case. Obstet. Gynec.
36:377-387, 1970.

NUMERICAL ANOMALIES

No attempt has been made to cover extensively the reports in this area. Instead a few select references, (admittedly controversial decisions had to be made), on the basis of priority, extensive review and critical evaluation of the data have been included. It is hoped that the reader will find other useful and important references in the reports included in this catalog.

01-

Kelly, S., Almy, R., Jakovic, L. and Buckner, L.: Autosomal monosomy in a spontaneous abortion. Lancet 1:166-167, 1965.
45,XX,-1.

02+

Honore, L. H., Dill, F. J. and Poland, B. J.: The association of hyadatidiform mole and trisomy 2. Obstet. Gynec. 43:232-237, 1974.

Lauritsen, J. G., Jonasson, J., Therkelsen, A. J., Lass, F., Lindsten, J. and Petersen, G. B.: Studies on spontaneous abortions. Fluorescence analysis of abnormal karyotypes. Hereditas 71:160-163, 1972.
47,XY,+2,Dp+,Gp-.

03-

Waxman, S. H., Arakaki, D. T. and Smith, J. B.: Cytogenetics of fetal abortions. Pediatrics 39:425-432, 1967.
Cases S-98 and S-25 in this report.
45,XX,-3.

03+

Carr, D. H.: Chromosome studies in spontaneous abortions. Obstet. Gynec. 26:308-326, 1965.
47,XX,+3.

Carr, D. H.: Chromosome anomalies as a cause of spontaneous abortion. Amer. J. Obstet. Gynec. 97:283-293, 1967.
47,X?,+3.

07+

Kuliev, A. M., Kukharenko, V. I., Grinberg, K. N., Vasileysky, S. S., Terskikh, V. V. and Stepanova, L. G.: Morhpological, autoradiographic, immunochemical and cytochemical investigation of a cell strain with trisomy 7 from a spontaneous abortus. Humangenetik 17:285-296, 1973.
47,XX,+7.
Cell strain LHC-162 was derived from an abortus received at the gestational age of 9 weeks from a 21 year old mother.

McCreanor, H. R., O'Malley, F. M. and Reid, R. A.: Trisomy in abortion material. Lancet 2:972-973, 1973.
47,XX,+7.

08+

Atkins, L., Holmes, L. B. and Riccardi, V. M.: Trisomy 8. J. Pediat. 84:302-304, 1974.

Bass, H. N. and Crandall, B. F.: Trisomy 8: An identifiable syndrome. Amer. J. Hum. Genet. 26:11A, 1974.
46,XX/47,XX,+8.
46,XY/47,XY,+8.

Bijlsma, J. B., Wijffels, J. C. H. M. and Tegelaers, W. H. H.: C8 trisomy mosaicism syndrome. Helv. Paediat. Acta 27:281-298, 1972.
47,XX and XY,+8.

Caspersson, T., Lindsten, J., Zech, L., Buckton, K. E. and Price, W. H.: Four patients with trisomy 8 identified by the fluorescence and Giemsa banding technique. J. Med. Genet. 9:1-7, 1972.
Trisomy 8 has been well delineated in this report.

de Grouchy, J., Jusso, F., Beguin, S., Turleau, C., Jalpert, P. and Laurent, C.: Blood clotting factor VII deficiency in three patients with trisomy 8. Ann. Genet. 17:105-108, 1974.
Cases 1 and 3 in this report.
46,XY/47,XY,+8.
Case 2 in this report.
47,XX,+8.

de Grouchy, J., Turleau, C. and Leonard, C.: Etude en fluorescence d'une trisomie C mosaique probablement 8: 46,XY/47,XY,?8+. Ann. Genet. 14:69-72, 1971.
46,XY/47,XX,?+8.

de la Chapelle, A.: Rotterdam Conference, 1974. Two of these cases were reported to have elevated levels of glutathione reductase, structural gene for which has been assigned on chromosome 8.

de la Chapelle, A., Schroder, J. and Vuopio, P.: 8-Trisomy in the bone marrow. Report of two cases. Clin. Genet. 3:470-476, 1972.
Case 1 in this report.
47,XY,+8.
Case 2 in this report.
47,XX,+8.
Both patients showed normal karyotypes in blood cultures and Case 2 had normal chromosomes in skin culture preparation as well.

Kakati, S., Nihill, M. and Sinha, A. K.: An attempt to establish trisomy 8 syndrome. Human-genetik 19:293-300, 1973.
47,XX,+8.

Lejeune, J. and Rethore, M. O.: Trisomies of chromosome No. 8. Nobel Symposium 23:214-216, 1973.
47,XX and XY,+8.
Descriptions for trisomies for short arm, and middle part and distal part of long arm can also be found in this report.

Riccardi, V. M., Greensher, A. and Lubs, H. A.: Trisomy 8: aneuploidy with diverse manifestations and causes. Amer. J. Hum. Genet. 26:72A, 1974.

Tuncbilek, E., Halicioglu, C. and Say, B.: Trisomy-8 syndrome. Humangenetik 23:23-29, 1974. 46,XY,+8/47,XY,+8.

Walravens, P. A., Greensher, A., Sparks, J. W. and Wesenberg, R. L.: Trisomy 8 mosaicism. Amer. J. Dis. Child. 128:564-566, 1974.

Wilson, M. G., Fujimoto, A. and Alfi, O. S.: Double autosomal trisomy and mosaicism for chromosome No. 8 and No. 21. J. Med. Genet. 11:96-101, 1974. 47,XX,+21/48,XX,+8,+21.

09+

Feingold, M. and Atkins, L.: A case of trisomy 9. J. Med. Genet. 10:184-187, 1973. Trisomy 9 in a patient who survived 28 days has been reported.

Haslam, R. H. A., Brooke, S. P., Moore, C. M., Thomas, G. H. and Neill, C. A.: Trisomy 9 mosaicism with multiple congenital anomalies. J. Med. Genet. 10:180-184, 1973.

Kurnick, J., Atkins, L., Feingold, M., Hills, J. and Dvorak, A.: Trisomy 9: predominance of cardiovascular, liver, brain, and skeletal anomalies in the first diagnosed case. Human Path. 5:223-232, 1974. An excellent record of autopsy findings in a 26 day old 47,XY,+9 infant.

10+

Nakagome, Y., Iinuma, K. and Matsui, I.: Trisomy 10 with mosaicism. A clinical and cytogenetic entity. Jap. J. Hum. Genet. 18:216-219, 1973. 46,XY/47,XY,+10.

Saint-Rome, G., Gagnon, J., Jelin, G. and Duhaime, M.: La trisomie C libre homogene et en mosaique. L'Union Medicale du Canada 101:2121-2129, 1972. 47,XX,+10. Two patients with a probable trisomy for chromosome 10 are described, one of which was a mosaic.

13+

Butler, L. J., Reiss, H. E., France, N. E. and Briddon, S.: Antenatal diagnosis of Patau's syndrome (trisomy 13) including a detailed pathological study of the fetus. J. Med. Genet. 10:367-370, 1973.

Lazjuk, G. J., Kravtsova, G. I., Kulazhenko, V. P., Yu, Usova, I. and Usoev, S. S.: Analysis of 137 cases of the trisomy D syndrome. Soviet Genetics 7:1338 and Genetika 7:116-129, 1971.

Patau, K., Smith, D. W., Therman, E., Inhorn, S. L. and Wagner, H. P.: Multiple congenital anomaly caused by an extra autosome. Lancet 1:790-793, 1960.
47,XX,+13.
D1 or 13 trisomy, also called Patau syndrome, was described in this report.

14+

Kajii, T., Ohama, K. and Ferrier, S. A.: Trisomy 14 in spontaneous abortus. Humangenetik 15:265-267, 1972.
47,XX,+14.

Kuliev, A. M., Kukharenko, V. I., Grinberg, K. N., Terskikh, V. V., Tamarkina, A. D., Bogomazov, E. A., Redkin, P. S. and Vasileysky, S. S.: Investigation of a cell strain with trisomy 14 from a spontaneously aborted human fetus. Humangenetik 21:1-12, 1974.
47,XY,+14.

Same entry as in 05q330 (Lucas and Wallace, 1972).

Murken, J. D., Bauchinger, M., Politzsch, D., Pfeifer, H., Suschke, J. and Haendle, H.: Trisomy D2 in a two and half years old girl (47,XX,14+). Humangenetik 10:254-268, 1970.
46,XX,+14.
Extra chromosome 14 identified by autoradiography, the clinical symptoms described appear to be different than those for trisomy 13.

15+

Same entry as in 15q000 (Bucher et al., 1973).

Same entry as in 15q210 (Howard, Stoddard and Yarbrough, 1974).

Lauritsen, J. G., Jonasson, J., Therkelsen, A. J., Lass, F., Lindsten, J. and Petersen, G. B.: Studies on spontaneous abortions. Fluorescence analysis of abnormal karyotypes. Hereditas 71:160-163, 1972.
47,XX and XY,+15.

Same entry as in 15q000 (Parker and Alfi, 1972).

16+

Carr, D. H.: Chromosome anomalies as a cause of spontaneous abortion. Amer. J. Obstet. Gynec. 97:283-293, 1967.
47,X?,+16.

Clendenin, T. M. and Benirschke, K.: Chromosome studies on spontaneous abortions. Laboratory Investigation 12:1281-1292, 1963.
Case No. 83 in this report.
47,XY,+16.
Also see
Benirschke, K.: Chromosomal studies on abortuses. New Eng. Obstet. Gynec. Soc. 17:171-183, 1963.

Dhadial, R. K., Machin, A. M. and Tait, S. M.: Chromosomal anomalies in spontaneously aborted human fetuses. Lancet 1:20-21, 1970.
47,XX or XY,+16.

Kyaosaar, M. E.: A cytogenetic study of spontaneous abortions. Genetika 8:158-160, 1972.
47,XY,+16.

Lauritsen, J. G., Jonasson, J., Therkelsen, A. J., Lass, F., Lindsten, J. and Petersen, G. B.: Studies on spontaneous abortions. Fluorescence analysis of abnormal karyotypes. Hereditas 71:160-163, 1972.
47,XX and XY,+16.

Same entry as in 0Yp110 (Lauritsen et al., 1972).

Taylor, A. I.:   Trisomy of chromosome 16 in a neonate.   47,XY,?16+.   J. Med. Genet. 8:123-125, 1971.
47,XY,?+16.

Waxman, S. H., Arakaki, D. T. and Smith, J. B.: Cytogenetics of fetal abortions.   Pediatrics 39:425-432, 1967.
Cases S-13, S-92 and S-163 in this report.
47,XX and XY,+16.
Case S-160 in this report.
46,XY/47,XY,+16.

18+

Atnip, R. L. and Summitt, R. L.:   Tetraploidy and 18-trisomy in a six-year-old triple mosaic boy. Cytogenetics 10:305-317, 1971.
46,XY/47,XY,+18/92,XXYY.

Same entry as in 130000 (Avirachan and Kajii, 1973).

Same entry as in 0X+, 18+, 48,XXY,+18 (Cohen and Bumbalo, 1967).

Crandall, B. F. and Ebbin, A. J.:   Trisomy 18 and 21 in two siblings.   Clin. Genet. 4:517-519, 1973.
47,XX,+18.
47,XX,+21.

Edwards, J. H., Harnden, D. G., Cameron, A. H., Crosse, V. M. and Wolff, O. H.:   A new trisomic syndrome.   Lancet 1:787-790, 1960.
47,XX,+18.
E1 or 18 trisomy, also called Edward syndrome, was first described in this report.
The extra chromosome was later interpreted as No. 18 instead of No. 17.

Same entry as in 0Yp110 (Lauritsen et al., 1972).

Ogita, S., Hasegawa, H., Matsumoto, M., Kamei, T., Shimamoto, T., Ohmishi, M. and Sugawa, T.: Prenatal diagnosis of E trisomy syndrome by

fetography. Obstet. Gynec. 43:887-892, 1974.
47,XY,+18.

Punnett, H. H.: 1973.
47,XX,+18.
Mutant Cell Repository No. GM-143.

Shibata, K., Waldenmaier, C. and Hirsch, W.: The
clinical and genetic picture of trisomy 18
(Edward's syndrome). Z. Kinderheilk. 116:13-22,
1973.
47,XY,+18.

Stoll, C., Levy, J. M. and Terrade, E.: Pro-
longed survival in trisomy 18. Ann. Pediat.
21:185-190, 1974.
47,XX,+18.
Karyotype confirmed by controlled heat denaturation technique was found in a 13 year old patient.

Same entry as in 0X- or 0Y- 45,X (Schinzel,
Schmid and Prader, 1974).

Surana, R. B., Bain, H. W. and Conen, P. E.: 18-
trisomy in a 15-year-old girl. Amer. J. Dis.
Child. 123:75-77, 1972.

20+

Same entry as in 14q000 (Krompotic et al., 1971).

21-

Al-Aish, M. S., de la Cruz, F., Goldsmith, A.,
Volpe, J., Mella, G. and Robinson, J. C.:
Autosomal monosomy in man. Complete monosomy G
(21-22) in a four and one half year old mentally
retarded girl. New Eng. J. Med. 277:777-784,
1967.
45,XX,21.
Extensive work-up was done on this case to rule
out mosaicism and translocation by the standard
(i.e., non-banding) techniques.

Klinger, H. P.:
45,XY,-21.
Mutant Cell Repository No. GM-137.

Mahoney, M.:
45,XX,-21.
Mutant Cell Repository No. GM-230.

Ohama, K. and Kajii, T.: Monosomy 21 in spontaneous abortus. Humangenetik 16:267-270, 1972.
45,XX,-21.

Weber, F. M., Sparkes, R. S. and Muller, H.: Double monosomy mosaicism (45,X/45,XX,21-) in a retarded child with multiple congenital malformations. Cytogenetics 10:404-412, 1971.
45,X/45,XX,-21.
This mosaic karyotype identified by quinacrine banding technique was described in a three year old girl with several anomalies.

21+

Same entry as in 0Yp110 (Baheux, Emerit and Roux, 1970).

Same entry as in 0Y0000 (Berger, Lejeune and Roy, 1973).

Caspersson, T., Hulten, M., Lindsten, J. and Zech, L.: Distinction between extra G-like chromosomes by quinacrine mustard fluorescence analysis. Exp. Cell Res. 63:240-243, 1970.
Chromosome 21 was found to be the one involved in Down syndrome by quinacrine banding pattern analyses.

Same entry as in 18+ (Crandall and Ebbin, 1973).

Same entry as in 02p110 (Creasy and Crolla, 1974).

Same entry as in 01p320 (de la Chapelle, 1973).

Same entry as in 0Yq100 (Genest, Bouchard and Bouchard, 1967).

Same entry as in 07q000 (Giraud et al., 1974).

Same entry as in 19p130 (Hamerton, Ray and

Douglas, 1973).

Same entry as in 21q110 (Hongell and Airaksinen, 1972).

Hsu, L. Y. F., Gertner, M., Leiter, E. and Hirschhorn, K.: Paternal trisomy 21 mosaicism and Down's syndrome. Amer. J. Hum. Genet. 23:592-601, 1971.

Kjessler, B. and de la Chapelle, A.: Meiosis and spermatogenesis in two postpubertal males with Down's syndrome: 47,XY,G+. Clin. Genet. 2:50-57, 1971.

Koch, G.: Down-syndrom. Mongolismus. Biblio-graphica Genetica Medica 1:1-283, 1973.
A useful bibliography of 1,754 articles on Down syndrome and related topics.

Same entry as in 010000 (Kontras et al., 1966).

Same entry as in 0Yq100 (Leisti, 1971).

Lejeune, J., Gautier, M. and Turpin, R.: Etude des chromosomes somatiques de neuf enfants mongoliens. C. R. Acad. Sci. 248:1721-1722, 1959.
47,XX and XY,+21.
Trisomy 21 condition was first described in this report in four girls and five boys.

Licznerski, G. and Lindsten, J.: Trisomy 21 in man due to maternal non-disjunction during the first meiotic division. Hereditas 70:153-154, 1972.

Same entry as in 02p100 (Lundsten, Vestermark and Philip, 1974).

Same entry as in 0Xq100 (Luthardt and Palmer, 1971).

Mellman, W. J.: 1974.
47,XY,+21.
Mutant Cell Repository No. GM-258.

Mikkelsen, M.: Down's syndrome. Current stage

of cytogenetic research. Humangenetik 12:1-28, 1971.

Same entry as in 02p100 (Miller et al., 1970).

Neu, R. L., Voorhees, M. L. and Gardner, L. I.: A case of 47,XX,(21q-)+ with some stigmata of Down's syndrome and an IQ of 77. J. Med. Genet. 8:528-529, 1971.
47,XX,del(21)(q).
47,XX,del(21)(pter to q:).

Newton, M. S., Cunningham, C., Jacobs, P. A., Price, W. H. and Fraser, I. A.: Chromosome survey of a hospital for the mentally subnormal. Part 2: Autosome abnormalities. Clin. Genet. 3:226-248, 1972.
M. R. C. Registry No. K67-209-66 in this report.
46,XY,+21,-13,-14,+der t(13q14q)mat.

Same entry as in 130000 (Newton et al., 1972).

Same entry as in 18p110 (Prieur et al., 1971).

Same entry as in 130000 (Scheres, 1972).

Same entry as in 130000 (Singh, Osborne and Horger, 1974).

Same entry as in 030000 (Soukup et al., 1969).

Same entry as in 0Yp110 (Sparkes, Muller and Veomett, 1970).

Same entry as in 03p140 (Subrt, 1974).

Same entry as in 03p000 (Subrt and Prchlikova, 1969).

Same entry as in 18q000 (Tenbrinck, 1974).

Same entry as in 21p130 (Uchida, 1973).

van der Hagen, C. B. and Berg, K.: Studies of human chromosomes by DNA-binding fluorochromes. II. Fluorescence characteristics of the supernumerary G chromosome in Down's syndrome. Clin. Genet. 2:58-60, 1971.

47,XX and XY,+21.
Extra chromosome identified as number 21 by fluorescence technique.

Vandevelde-Staquet, M. F., Breynaert, R., Wal-baum, R., Saint-Aubert, P., Farriaux, J. P. and Fontaine, G.: La descendance des meres trisomi-ques 21 (A propos d'une observation). J. Genet. Hum. 21:187-206, 1973.
A phenotypically normal (except hypospadias) 46,XY child born to a 47,XX,+21 woman is reported along with a review of previously reported offspring born to mothers with Down syndrome (total of 21 cases).

Same entry as in 190000 (Vogel and Loning, 1973).

Same entry as in 13q120 (von Koskull and Aula, 1974).

Same entry as in 08+ (Wilson, Fujimoto and Alfi, 1974).

Zergollern, L., Hoefnagel, D., Benirschke, K. and Corcoran, P. A.: A patient with trisomy 21 and a reciprocal translocation in the 13/15 group. Cytogenetics 3:148-158, 1964.
45,XY,t(DqDq).
45,XX and XY,der t(DqDq)pat.
Propositus D. B. in this report.
45,XY,der t(DqDq)pat,+21.

Zeuthen, E., Nielsen, J. and Nielsen, A.: Prevalence of Down's syndrome. Hereditas 75:136-137, 1973.
Discussion on the prevalence of the condition in Denmark.

22-

DeCicco, F., Steele, M. W., Pan, S. F. and Park, S. C. P.: Monosomy of chromosome no. 22: a case report. J. Pediat. 83:836-838, 1973.
45,XX,-22.

Same entry as in 22p100 (Stoll, Rohmer and Sauvage, 1973).

22+

Bass, H. N., Crandall, B. F. and Sparkes, R. S.:
Probable trisomy 22 identified by fluorescent and
trypsin-Giemsa banding. Ann. Genet. 16:189-192,
1973.
Patient TSC 021262 in this report.
47,XX,+22.

Buhler, E. M., Mehes, K., Muller, H. and Stalder,
G. R.: Cat-eye syndrome, a partial trisomy 22.
Humangenetik 15:150-162, 1972.
47,XY,+22q-.

Same entry as in 22q100 (Buhler et al., 1972).

Goodman, R. M., Katznelson, M. B. M., Spero, M.,
Shaki, R., Padeh, B. and Sodan, N.: The question
of trisomy 22 syndrome. J. Pediat. 79:174-175,
1971.
47,XY,+22.

Hirschhorn, K., Lucas, M. and Wallace, I.:
Precise identification of various chromosomal
abnormalities. Ann. Hum. Genet. 36:375-379,
1973.
Family C(GC 785) in this report.
47,XX,+22.

Hsu, L. Y. F., Shapiro, L. R., Gertner, M.,
Lieber, E. and Hirschhorn, K.: Trisomy 22: a
clinical entity. J. Pediat. 79:12-19, 1971.

Punnett, H. H., Kistenmacher, M. L., Toro-sola,
M. A. and Kohn, G.: Quinacrine fluorescence and
Giemsa banding in trisomy 22. Theo. Appl. Genet.
43:134-138, 1973.

MAR+

Armendares, S., Buentello, L. and Salamanca, F.:
An extra small metacentric autosome in a mentally
retarded boy with multiple malformations. J.
Med. Genet. 8:378-380, 1971.
47,XY,+mar.

Borgaonkar, D. S.: Application of new technics
of chromosome identification to cytogenetic

problems. Birth Defects: Original Article Series
9 No. 1:171-182, 1973.
47,XY,+mar.
The problem of identifying a small, extra chromosome is discussed.

Same entry as in 17p100 (Borgaonkar, McKusick and
Farber, 1973).

Borgaonkar, D. S., Schimke, R. N. and Thomas, G.
H.: Report of five unrelated patients with a
small, metacentric, extra chromosome or fragment.
J. Genet. Hum. 19:207-222, 1971.
46,XX and XY,+mar.

Finley, W. H., Finley, S. C. and Monsky, D.: An
extra small metacentric chromosome in association
with multiple congenital abnormalities. J. Med.
Genet. 8:381-383, 1971.
47,XX,+mar.

Freedom, R. M. and Gerald, P. S.: Congenital
cardiac disease and the "cat-eye" syndrome.
Amer. J. Dis. Child. 126:16-18, 1973.
47,XX and XY,+mar.

Friedrich, U. and Nielsen, J.: Bisatellited
extra small metacentric chromosome in newborns.
Clin. Genet. 6:23-31, 1974.
Proband Nos. 4767, 6013 and 9421 in this report.
47,XX and XY,+mar.
47,XX and XY,+der(mar)mat.

Fryns, J. P., Eggermont, E., Verresen, H. and van
den Berghe, H.: A newborn with the cat-eye
syndrome. Humangenetik 15:242-248, 1972.
Patient G. B. in this report.
46,XY,/47,XY,+mar.

Same entry as in 15q210 (Howard, Stoddard and
Yarbrough, 1974).

Same entry as in 17q110 (Latta and Hoo, 1974).

Same entry as in 07p100 (Noel et al., 1973).

0X-   or 0Y-   -   45,X

Alexander, D., Ehrhardt, A. A. and Money, J. W.: Defective figure drawing, geometric and human, in Turner's syndrome. J. Nerv. Ment. Dis. 142:161-167, 1966.

Anderson, H., Filipsson, R., Fluur, E., Koch, B., Lindsten, J. and Wedenberg, E.: Hearing impairment in Turner's syndrome. Acta Oto-Laryngologica Suppl. 247:1-26, 1969.

Ehrhardt, A. A., Greenberg, N. and Money, J. W.: Female gender identity and absence of fetal gonadal hormones: Turner's syndrome. Johns Hopk. Med. J. 126:237-248, 1970.

Ferguson-Smith, M. A., Alexander, D. S., Bowen, P., Goodman, R. M., Kaufmann, B. N., Jones, H. W. and Heller, R. H.: Clinical and cytogenetical studies in female gonadal dysgenesis and their bearing on the cause of Turner's syndrome. Cytogenetics 3:355-383, 1964.

Ford, C. E., Polani, P. E., Briggs, J. H. and Bishop, P. M. F.: A presumptive human XXY/XX mosaic. Nature 183:1030-1032, 1959.
In an addendum to the paper the authors cited a single case of Turner syndrome as having 45 chromosomes, was chromatin negative, and XO constitution.
45,X.

Ford, C. E., Jones, K. W., Polani, P. E., de Almeida, J. C. C. and Briggs, J. H.: A sex-chromosome anomaly in a case of gonadal dysgenesis (Turner's syndrome). Lancet 1:711-713, 1959.
45,X was first described in this report.

Money, J. W.: Cytogenetic and psychosexual incongruities with a note on space-form blindness. Amer. J. Psychiat. 119:820-827, 1963.

Money, J. W.: Two cytogenetic syndromes: psychologic comparisons. I. Intelligence and specific-factor quotients. J. Psychiat. Res. 2:223-231, 1964.

Price, W. H., Lauder, I. J. and Wilson, J.: The electrocardiogram and sex chromosome aneuploidy.

Clin. Genet. 6:1-14, 1974.
"It is confirmed that in 47,XYY males the atrio-
ventricular conduction is delayed and that in
45,X females it is accelerated".

Schinzel, A., Schmid, W. and Prader, A.: Turner
phenotype: Mosaic 45,X/47,XY,+18. J. Med. Genet.
11:101-104, 1974.

OX+   -   47,XXX

Barr, M. L., Sergovich, F. R., Carr, D. H. and
Shaver, E. L.: The triple-X female: An appraisal
based on a study of 12 cases and a review of the
literature.   Canad. Med. Ass. J. 101:247-258,
1969.

Same entry as in OX+ 18+ -   48,XXX,+18 (Emberger,
Sarran and Balzing, 1971).

Jacobs, P. A., Baikie, A. G., Court Brown, W. M.,
MacGregor, T. N., MacLean, N. and Harnden, D. G.:
Evidence for the existence of the human "super
female." Lancet 2:423-425, 1959.
47,XXX was first described in this report.

Klinger, H. P.:   1973.
47,XXX.
Mutant Cell Repository No. GM-254.

Olanders, S.:   Double Barr bodies in women in
mental hospitals.   Brit. J. Psychiat. 113:1097-
1099, 1967.

Telfer, M. A., Richardson, C. E., Helmken, J. and
Smith, G. F.: Divergent phenotypes among 48,XXXX
and 47,XXX females. Amer. J. Hum. Genet. 22:326-
335, 1970.

OX+ - 48,XXXX

Gardner, R. J. M., Veale, A. M. O., Sands, V. E.
and Holdaway, M. D. H.: XXXX syndrome: case
report, and a note on genetic counselling and
fertility. Humangenetik 17:323-330, 1973.
Reportedly cited as a 19th case with this karyotype.   A table of characteristics and parental
ages has been provided on these cases.

Pena, S. B., Ray, M., Douglas, G., Loadman, E. and Hamerton, J. L.: A 48,XXXX female. J. Med. Genet. 11:211-215, 1974.

Same entry as in 0X+ 47,XXX (Telfer et al., 1970).

Tumba, A., Timmerman, J., Fryns, J. P. and van den Berghe, H.: A newborn with 48,XXXX karyotype. Case report and review of the literature. Ann. Pediat. In press, 1974.

Wagenbichler, von P., Golob, E. and Szilvassy, J.: Ein falle von X-tetrasomie (48,XXXX). Klin. Wschr. 85:5-10, 1973.

Walbaum, R., Vandevelde-Staquet, M. F., Lefebre, Ch., Gramey, D. K., DeLattve B. and LeConte, D.: Syndrome 48,XXXX chez un nourrisson. J. Genet. Hum. 21:43-56, 1973.

0X+ - 49,XXXXX

Berger, R., Loewe-Lyon, S., Derre, J. and Ortiz, M. A.: Syndrome 49,XXXXX. J. Pediat. 20:965-967, 1973.

Brody, J., Fitzgerald, M. G. and Spiers, A. S. D.: A female child with five X chromosomes. J. Pediat. 70:105-109, 1967.

0X+ - 47,XXY

Same entry as in 0Xq200 (Chandra et al., 1971).

Same entry as in 08q000 (Chen and Woolley, 1971).

Same entry as in 09q000 (Dumars, Reed and Lawce, 1974).

Hook, E. B.: Racial differentials in the prevalence rates of males with sex chromosome abnormalities (XXY, XYY) in security settings in the United States. Amer. J. Hum. Genet. 26:504-511, 1974.

Same entry as in 0Yp110 (Jacobs and Ross, 1966).

Jacobs, P. A. and Strong, J. A.: A case of human intersexuality having a possible XXY sex-determining mechanism. Nature 183:302-303, 1959.
47,XXY.
This chromosome constitution was first described by these authors in a clinical condition commonly referred as Klinefelter syndrome but it was not cited as such by the authors of this report.

Same entry as in 13p100 (Lindenbaum, Blackwell and de Sa, 1972).

Same entry as in 0Yq100 (Miller et al., 1967).

Same entry as in 0X- or 0Y- - 45,X (Money, 1964).

Palutke, W. A., Chen, Y. and Chen, H.: Presence of brightly fluorescent material in testes of XX males. J. Med. Genet. 10:170-174, 1973.

Wahrman, J., Berant, M., Jacobs, J., Aviad, I. and Ben-hur, N.: The oral-facial-digital syndrome: A male-lethal condition in a boy with 47/XXY chromosomes. Pediatrics 37:812-821, 1966.

Same entry as in 0X0000 (Zang et al., 1969).

0X+ - 48,XXXY

Ferguson-Smith, M. A., Johnston, A. W. and Handmaker, S. D.: Primary amentia and micro-orchidism associated with an XXXY sex-chromosome constitution. Lancet 2:126-128, 1960.

Ferrier, P. E., Ferrier, S. A. and Pescia, G.: The XXXY Klinefelter syndrome in childhood. Amer. J. Dis. Child. 127:104-105, 1974.
The authors have attempted to delineate the phenotype of 48,XXXY males with an objective of diagnosing the condition before puberty.

Simpson, J. L., Morillo-Cucci, G., Horwith, M., Stiefel, F. H., Feldman, F. and German, J.: Abnormalities of human sex chromosomes. VI. Monozygotic twins with the complement 48,XXXY. Humangenetik 21:301-308, 1974.

Vormittag, W. and Weninger, M.: XXXY Klinefelter's syndrome. Humangenetik 15:327-333, 1972.

OX+ - 49,XXXXY

Aronsson, S., Lindgren, F. and Svanstrom, L.: Two cases of the sex chromosome aberration XXXXY. Hereditas 55:126-128, 1966.

Assemany, S. R., Neu, R. L. and Gardner, L. I.: XXXXY syndrome in a phenotypic male infant with associated cardiac abnormalities. Humangenetik 12:101-104, 1971.

Boon, W. H. and Seng, T. C.: A Chinese infant with XXXXY sex chromosomes. J. Singapore Paediat. Soc. 12:52-57, 1970.

Christensen, M. F. and Therkelsen, A. J.: A case of the XXXXY chromosome anomaly with four maternal X chromosomes and diabetic glucose tolerance. Acta Paediat. Scand. 59:706-710, 1970.

Cunningham, M. D. and Ragsdale, J. L.: Genital anomalies of an XXXXY male subject. J. Urol. 107:872-874, 1972.

Same entry as in 04q350 (de la Chapelle and Schroder, 1973).

Farquhar, H. G. and Walker, S.: An XXXXY chromosome abnormality. Ann. Hum. Genet. 28:11-19, 1964.

Fraccaro, M., Kayser, K. and Lindsten, J.: A child with 49 chromosomes. Lancet 2:899-902, 1960.

Galindo, J. and Baar, H. S.: The XXXXY sex chromosome abnormality. Arch. Dis. Child. 41:82-86, 1966.

Gardner, R. J. M., Sands, V. E., Veale, A. M. O., Howarth, D. A. and Parslow, M. I.: XXXXY syndrome with mosaicism: case report. New Zealand Med. J. 76:22-27, 1972.

Murken, J. D. and Scholz, W.: Serologische

klarung der Herkunft der uberzahligen X-chromo-
somen beim XXXXY-syndrom. Blut 16:164-168, 1968.
49,XXXXY.
On the basis of Xga blood group characteristic
[father Xg(a+), mother Xg(a-), and the boy Xg(a-
)] it was concluded that the boy must have
received all of his four X chromosomes from his
mother.

Same entry as in 04q350 (Ockey and de la Chapelle, 1967).

Rerrick, E. G.: Klinefelter's syndrome variant,
XXXX/XXXXY mosaic. J. Maine Med. Ass. 60:90-93,
1969.

Sacrez, R., Clavert, J., Kleir, M., Paira, M.,
Rumpler, J., Mandry, J. and Meyer, R.: Dysgene-
sie gonado-somatique XXXXY. Arch. Franc. Pediat.
22:41-52, 1965.

See, G., Dayras, J. U., Hartmann, O. and Proffit,
M.: A new case of 49,XXXXY dysgenesis. Sem. des
Hop. Paris 50:229-232, 1974.

Siniscalo, M.: Personal Communication, 1974.
Mutant Cell Repository No. GM-326.

Terheggen, H. G., Pfeiffer, F. A., Haug, H.,
Hertl, M., Diggins, A. and Schunke, W.: The
XXXXY syndrome. Report of 7 new cases and review
of the literature. Z. Kinderheilk. 115:209-233,
1973.

Tumba, A.: Le phenotype XXXXY: etude analytique
et synthetique a propos de trois cas personnels
et de 67 autres case de la literature. J. Genet.
Hum. 20:9-48, 1972.

Wong, H. B. and Chua, T. S.: A Chinese infant
with XXXXY sex chromosomes. J. Singapore Paediat. Soc. 12:52-57, 1970.

Zaleski, W. A., Houston, C. S., Pozsonyi, J. and
Ying, K. L.: The XXXXY chromosome anomaly:
report of three new cases and review of 30 cases
from the literature. Canad. Med. Ass. J.
94:1143-1154, 1966.

OY+ - 47,XYY

Borgaonkar, D. S. and Shah, S. A.: The XYY
chromosome male - or syndrome? Prog. Med.
Genet. 10:135-222, 1974.

Same entry as in +OX 47,XXY (Hook, 1974).

Money, J. W., Annecillo, C., van Orman, B. and
Borgaonkar, D. S.: Cytogenetics, hormones and
behavior disability: comparison of XYY and XXY
syndromes. Clin. Genet., in press, 1974.

Same entry as in OX- or OY- 45,X (Price, Lauder
and Wilson, 1974).

Sandberg, A. A., Koepf, G. F., Ishihara, T. and
Hauschka, T. S.: An XYY human male. Lancet
2:488-489, 1961.

OY+ - 48,XYYY

Ridler, M. A. C., Lax, R., Mitchell, M. J.,
Shapiro, J. and Saldana-Garcia, P.: An adult
male with XYYY sex chromosomes. Clin. Genet.
4:69-77, 1973.

OY+ - 49,XYYYY

van den Berghe, H., Verresen, H. and Cassiman, J.
J.: A male with 4 Y-chromosomes. J. Clin.
Endocr. 28:1370-1372, 1968.
45,X/49,XYYYY mosaic.
A fifteen year old boy was studied.

OX+ 18+ - 48,XXX,+18

Emberger, J. M., Sarran, R. and Balzing, P.: A
case of double trisomy: 48,XXX,18+. Ann. Genet.
17:301-303, 1971.

Haas, L. and Lewis, F. J. W.: Double trisomy:
Trisomy 17-18 with triple X in a female infant.
J. Pediat. 69:660-662, 1966.

OX+ 18+ - 48,XXY,+18

Cohen, M. M. and Bumbalo, T. S.: Double aneup-

loidy.   Trisomy-18 and Klinefelter's syndrome.
Amer. J. Dis. Child. 113:483-486, 1967.

OX+   21+ -   48,XXY,+21

Erdtmann, B., Gomes de Freitas, A. A., de Souza,
R. P. and Salzano, F. M.: Klinefelter's syndrome
and G trisomy. J. Med. Genet. 8:364-368, 1971.

Ford, C. E., Jones, K. W., Miller, O. J., Mitt-
woch, U., Penrose, L. S., Ridler, M. A. C. and
Shapiro, A.:   The chromosomes in a patient
showing both mongolism and the Klinefelter
syndrome. Lancet 1:709-710, 1959.

Hecht, F., Nievaard, J. E., Duncanson, N.,
Miller, J. R., Higgins, J. V., Kimberling, W. J.,
Walker, F. A., Smith, G. S., Thuline, H. C. and
Tischler, B.:   Double aneuploidy: The frequency
of XXY in males with Down's syndrome. Amer. J.
Hum. Genet. 21:352-359, 1969.

OY+ 21+ - 48,XYY, +21

Osztovics, M., Ivady, G. and Buhler, E. M.: XYY
chromosomal complement, proven by fluorescence,
in a child with trisomy 21: 48,XYY,21+. Humangenetik 13:144-150, 1971.

Verresen, H. and van den Berghe, H.: Trisomy 21
and XYY. Lancet 1:609, 1965.
This double aneuploidy was first described in
this report.

OX+ OY+ - 48,XXYY

Borgaonkar, D. S., Mules, E. and Char, F.: Do
the 48,XXYY males have a characteristic phenotype? - A review. Clin. Genet. 1:272-293, 1970.

Muldal, S. and Ockey, C. H.: The "double male":
a new chromosome constitution in Klinefelter's
syndrome. Lancet 2:492-493, 1960.

Singer, H., Zankl, H. and Rodewald-Rudescu, A.:
Combined Klinefelter-Down syndrome or XXYY
syndrome? Humangenetik 19:261-264, 1973.

OX+   OY+ -   49,XXXYY

Bray, P. and Josephine, A.: An XXXYY sex-chromosome anomaly.   Report of a mentally deficient
male. JAMA 184:179-182, 1963.

Lecluse-van der Britt, F. A., Hagemeijer, A.,
Smit, E. M. E., Visser, H. K. A. and Vaandrager,
G. J.:   An infant with an XXXYY karyotype. Clin.
Genet. 5:263-270, 1974.

OX+   OY+ -   49,XXYYY

Gracey, M. and Fitzgerald, M. G.: The XXYYY sex
chromosome complement in a mentally retarded
child. Australian Paediat. J. 3:119-121, 1967.

POLYPLOIDY: Selected recent references are listed
here.   Reference to earlier reports can be found
in these.

Same entry as in 18+ (Atnip and Summitt, 1971).

Kuliev, A. M.: Relationship between anomalies of
phenotype and karyotype in human embryogenesis.
Genetika 8:140-153, 1972.

Niebuhr, E.:   Triploidy in man. Cytogenetical
and clinical aspects. Humangenetik 21:103-125,
1974.

Uchida, I. A. and Lin, C. C.: Identification of
triploid genome by fluorescence microscopy.
Science 176:304-305, 1972.

Weaver, D. D. and Gartler, S. M.: Evidence for
two active X chromosomes in a human triploid
line. Amer. J. Hum. Genet. 26:91A, 1974.

CHROMOSOMAL BREAKAGE SYNDROMES

In this section of the catalog I have included those disorders in which generalized chromosomal anomalies have been described. These disorders will be listed alphabetically and a few selected references for each will also be listed alphabetically. Further details regarding their mode of inheritance and phenotypic manifestations can be found in McKusick's Mendelian Inheritance in Man. The term 'Chromosomal Breakage Syndromes' was coined by Dr. Victor A. McKusick in 1968 (Birth Defects: Original Article Series V(5); 1969) while planning The First Conference on The Clinical Delineation of Birth Defects. Part V. Phenotypic Aspects of Chromosomal Aberrations (German, 1969). The chromosomal anomalies are not restricted to or peculiar to any one particular chromosome. They were, therefore, not listed in the first two sections of the catalog.

German, J.: Chromosomal breakage syndromes. Birth Defects: Original Article Series V(5):117-131, 1969.

Ataxia-telangiectasia (or Louis-Bar syndrome).

Hecht, F., McCaw, B. K. and Koler, R. D.: Ataxia-telangiectasia-clonal growth of translocation lymphocytes. New Eng. J. Med. 289:286-291, 1973.

Hecht, F., Koler, R. D., Rigas, D. A., Dahnke, G. S., Case, M. P., Tisdale, V. and Miller, R. W.: Leukaemia and lymphocytes in ataxia-telangiectasia. Lancet 2:1193, 1966.

Rary, J. M., Bender, M. A. and Kelly, T. E.: Cytogenetic studies of ataxia-telangiectasia. Amer. J. Hum. Genet. 26:70A, 1974.

Bloom syndrome

German, J.: Bloom's syndrome. I. Clinical and genetical observations in the first 27 patients. Amer. J. Hum. Genet. 21:196-227, 1969.

German, J.: Chromosomal breakage in a rare and probably genetically determined syndrome of man. Science 148:506-507, 1965.

Sawitsky, A., Bloom, D. and German, J.: Chromosomal breakage and acute leukemia in congenital telangiectatic erythema and stunted growth. Ann. Intern. Med. 65:487-495, 1966.

Fanconi anemia

Swift, M. R. and Hirschhorn, K.: Fanconi's anemia. Inherited susceptibility to chromosome breakage in various tissues. Ann. Intern. Med. 65:496-503, 1966.

de Grouchy, J., de Nava, C., Marchand, J. C., Feingold, J. and Turleau, C.: Cytogenetic and biochemical studies of eight cases of Fanconi's anemia. Ann. Genet. 15:29-40, 1972.

Incontinentia pigmenti

Cantu, J. M., del Castillo, V., Jiminez, M. and Ruiz-Barquin, E.: Chromosomal instability in incontinentia pigmenti. Ann. Genet. 16:117-119, 1973.

de Grouchy, J., Bonnette, J., Brussieux, J., Roidot, M. and Begin, P.: Cassures chromosomiques dans l'incontinentia pigmenti. Etude d'une famille. Ann. Genet. 15:61, 1972.

Scleroderma

Emerit, I. and Housset, E.: Chromosome studies on bone marrow from patients with systemic sclerosis. Evidence for chromosomal breakage in vivo. Biomedicine 19:550-554, 1973.

Emerit, I., Levy, A. and Housset, E.: Chromosomal breakage in scleroderma. Possible presence of a breakage factor in the serum of patients. Ann. Genet. 16:135-138, 1973.

Xeroderma pigmentosum

Cleaver, J. E.: Defective repair replication of

DNA in Xeroderma pigmentosum. Nature 218:652-656, 1968.

Cleaver, J. E.: Xeroderma pigmentosum. Progress and regress. J. Invest. Dermat. 60:374-380, 1973.

AUTHOR INDEX

222

SELECTED SYNDROME SUBJECT INDEX